AIDS

A Strategy for Nursing Care

Robert J. Pratt

RN, BA, MSc, RGN, STD (Lond), DipN (Lond)

Head of Department of Continuing Education
Charing Cross School of Nursing
London

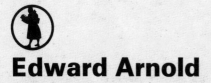

Edward Arnold

© Robert J. Pratt 1986

First published in Great Britain 1986 by
Edward Arnold (Publishers) Ltd, 41 Bedford Square, London WC1B 3DQ

Edward Arnold (Australia) Pty Ltd, 80 Waverley Road, Caulfield East,
Victoria 3145, Australia

Edward Arnold, 3 East Read Street, Baltimore, Maryland 21202, U.S.A.

Reprinted 1987

British Library Cataloguing in Publication Data

Pratt, Robert J.
    AIDS : a strategy for nursing care.
    1. AIDS (Disease) —— Patients
    I. Title
    362.1'9697   RC607.A26

    ISBN 0-7131-4517-X

Text set in 10/11 pt Times Compugraphic
by Colset Private Limited, Singapore
Printed and bound in Great Britain by Richard Clay Ltd.

I am indebted to Evangeline A. Karn, Senior Tutor, Department of
Continuing Education at Charing Cross School of Nursing, for her patient
proofreading and advice on style.

Contents

Introduction

> In the face of intense and immediate crisis, when an outbreak of
> plague implanted fear of imminent death in an entire community,
> ordinary routines and customary restraints broke down. Rituals
> arose to discharge anxiety and local panic often provoked bizarre
> behavior. The first efforts at ritualizing responses to the plague took
> extreme and ugly forms.
>
> *Plagues and Peoples*. W.H. McNeill.

Shortly before Christmas in 1981, the first patient with AIDS in the
United Kingdom lay dying in a London hospital. Medical and nursing
experts, casting a nervous glance at the United States where over three
hundred cases of this new disease had been identified, probably knew
from the beginning that the UK would not escape this developing
epidemic.

As 1982 and 1983 came and went, more cases were seen and, in a
sense, our worst fears were realised. Cases of AIDS were no longer
being imported into the UK but rather, we had our own endemic brand,
which was quickly spreading. Certain aspects of this particular disease
were especially alarming; its cause was unknown as was its means of
spread. Treatment of the various infections and cancers seen in this disease was ineffective, no–one surviving once the disease took hold.
Almost all of the affected were young adults, mostly men, and fear of
the disease became a parallel epidemic in its own right.

The heady months of 1984 brought both good news and bad news.
Brilliant research work by French scientists the year before had
uncovered the causative agent of AIDS. This was now confirmed by
researchers in America. With this discovery, the different ways in which
the epidemic was spreading also became clear and it seemed only a
matter of time before a vaccine would be available to stop, once and for
all, this ferocious disease. Nurses, however, noticed that increasing
numbers of patients, either with AIDS or under investigation for AIDS-
related conditions, continued to be admitted, and, thanks to the
hysteria and panic whipped up by a sensation-seeking media, health

care workers became as confused and frightened as everyone else. As always, the twenty-four hour care of these patients, like all other patients, was the paramount responsibility of nurses and they often seemed surrounded by frightened and sometimes hostile ancillary staff; domestics refusing to clean patients' rooms, catering staff refusing to serve meal trays to patients with AIDS, porters refusing to transport patients with this disease and undertakers refusing to accept the bodies of patients who had died from AIDS. Even some medical staff, (notably surgeons), would refuse to treat patients who had AIDS. Draconian infectious disease control procedures, bearing no logical relationship to the known facts of transmission, were often implemented, regardless of cost either in nursing time or in the further, deepening sense of isolation of these patients, frightened of becoming ever more abandoned.

In 1985, 165 new cases brought the total number of individuals in the UK with AIDS to 273. The Communicable Disease Surveillance Centre suggested that as the numbers continued to increase, in 1988, 2000 new cases might reasonably be expected[1].

This year also saw the introduction of a blood test which could detect previous exposure to the AIDS virus. This test showed that not all individuals infected with the AIDS virus went on to develop AIDS; others developed a less severe illness as a consequence of infection. Many remained healthy, free of any clinical symptoms, but *infected and infectious*. The Chief Medical Officer for the Department of Health and Social Security estimated that there might be over 10 000 such individuals in the UK (estimates of asymptomatic infected individuals in the USA ranged from 500 000 to one and a half million)[2]. Not only were these large numbers of infected individuals now able to escalate the epidemic dramatically, but also suspicion grew that these thousands of asymptomatic carriers might not remain asymptomatic as the years went by. It was known by 1985 that the AIDS virus not only attacked the immune system, but also attacked cells in the brain, leading, in many cases, to dementia[3]. It seemed reasonable to speculate that everyone infected with this virus would eventually suffer some form of ill health as a consequence. No health care system, in any part of the world, including the National Health Service in the UK, seemed prepared for even the present number of cases of people with fully expressed AIDS. How they would cope with the 'worst case' scenario of caring for increased numbers of currently asymptomatic infected individuals was not a pleasant thought to contemplate.

By 1986, there was not the least doubt that AIDS and AIDS-related conditions posed the most significant public health issue of our time. Not only were there the American and European epidemics, but major epidemics were also occurring in Central Africa, South America and in

Australia. AIDS had become of truly pandemic proportions. It was clear that it would be with us, in our hospitals and in our communities for years to come.

Dealing with the disease one day at a time, and one patient at a time, professional nurses have built up considerable expertise in developing individualized nursing care strategies, designed to deliver compassionate, non-judgemental, efficient and effective nursing care to large numbers of relatively young people, suffering and dying in fear and confusion. It is the nurse who cares for these patients. This text has been written to provide guidance and support, to share collective expertise, to reassure and to inform. Like our predecessors in the great epidemics of the past, nurses must be brave in the face of this current epidemic. We cannot abandon any of our patients, nor would we wish to do so. With accurate information, planned nursing care can be designed to safely and competently meet the needs of patients suffering from one of the most devastating diseases seen in recent times. On the eve of World War II, the American President, Franklin D. Roosevelt, told the American people, '. . . we have nothing to fear except fear itself.' For health care workers confronting the calamity of AIDS in the 1980s, the same is equally true. The enemy is not only the AIDS virus, but equally, fear, ignorance and prejudice. If in a small way this text neutralizes some of these factors, it will have been worth the effort.

References

1. Acheson, E.D. (1985). The CMO's briefing on AIDS. *THS Health Summary*. 2(VIII) August, pp 6–7
2. Acheson, E.D. (1986). AIDS: A challenge for the public health. *Lancet*. i(8482), March 22, pp 662–6
3. Sattaur, O. More evidence for brain disease in AIDS. *New Scientist*. 10 October 1985, p 26

1

The Evolving Epidemic

> The Plague had swallowed up everything and everyone. No longer were there individual destinies, only a collective destiny, made of plague and the emotions shared by all. Strongest of these emotions was the sense of exile and of deprivation, with all the cross-currents of revolt and fear set up by these.
>
> *The Plague*. Albert Camus

In the early months of 1981, five young men were admitted to various hospitals in Los Angeles, suffering from an unusual type of pneumonia caused by a commonly occurring protozoa known as *Pneumocystis carinii*. Previously, pneumonia caused by *P. carinii* had only been seen in patients who were immunocompromised, such as infants born with a primary immune deficiency (e.g. severe combined immune deficiency – 'SCID') or in adults whose immune system became deficient due to other causes, i.e. secondary immune deficiency states. Most cases of pneumonia caused by *P. carinii* had been observed in renal transplant units where patients had received immuno-suppressant chemotherapy following kidney transplants, or in oncology units, where patients had been immuno-suppressed as a result of receiving anti-cancer chemotherapy. Most individuals have been exposed to this microbe and it is part of the normal flora of many people. In individuals with a competent immune system it is harmless. Only in individuals with a faulty immune system can it cause disease, in which case the treatment of choice was a little-used antibiotic manufactured in the United Kingdom known as pentamidine isethionate. The physician in charge of the five cases in Los Angeles was puzzled. These five patients were all young men, who had evidence of a widespread immunodeficiency without any apparent reason. They had evidence of other infections and, coincidentally, they were all homosexual. The Communicable Disease Center ('CDC') in Atlanta, Georgia, was notified and supplies of pentamidine were requested, although by this time, two of the five patients had died. The CDC, which has as part of its function the task of monitoring the trend of infectious diseases throughout the United States and its territories, published an account of these five cases in its weekly bulletin, the *Morbidity and Mortality Weekly Report* (MMWR) on 5 June, 1981 and noted that the occurrence of pneumonia caused by *P. carinii* ('pneumocystosis') in five previously healthy individuals, who had no known reason for their defective immune status, was unusual, and questioned whether their homosexual lifestyle, or a disease acquired through sexual contact, could be associated with the development of the defects in the immune system which led to pneumocystosis[1].

Probably then no-one actually suspected the magnitude of the epidemic that was in the making. However, evidence of the gathering storm was soon starting to arrive.

At about the same time as physicians in Los Angeles had reported the cluster of cases of pneumocystosis, physicians in New York City notified the CDC of the occurrence of a severe form of Kaposi's sarcoma in 26 young men. Kaposi's sarcoma is a vascular neoplasm, uncommon in the United States and in Western Europe, being seen mainly in elderly men where it is manifested by skin lesions and a chronic clinical course (mean survival time is 8–13 years). However, in 1978 Kaposi's sarcoma had been described in patients who had undergone renal transplants and had received immunosuppressant therapy and in others who were iatrogenically immunosuppressed.

Of the 26 patients reported to the CDC in July of 1981, all had evidence of an immunodeficiency not related to any known cause, and several had other serious infections (four having pneumocystosis). All were homosexual[2].

Simultaneously, an additional 10 cases of pneumocystosis in healthy young gay men in Los Angeles and San Francisco were reported, two of whom also had Kaposi's sarcoma. All these patients had evidence of immunodeficiency with no known underlying cause. The following month saw an additional 70 cases of these two conditions[3]. It was then clear that an epidemic was brewing. This was an epidemic in which death would be caused by one or more unusual, opportunistic infections or by cancer, present only because the immune system had broken down due to unknown reasons.

Extremely alarmed, the CDC instituted a nation-wide surveillance programme in July 1981. The new disease was termed the *Acquired Immune Deficiency Syndrome* and it was characterized as the occurrence of unusual infections or cancers in previously healthy individuals, due to an immunodeficiency of unknown cause. The surveillance definition of AIDS is described in Table 1.1.

Table 1.1   Surveillance definition of AIDS – 1982[4]

The presence of a reliably diagnosed disease at least moderately predictive of cellular immune deficiency and the absence of an underlying cause for the immune deficiency or of any defined cause for reduced resistance to the disease.

Diseases at least moderately predictive of cellular immune deficiency

A.   Cancers
   1. Kaposi's sarcoma
   2. Primary lymphoma of brain
B.   Protozoal and helminthic infections
   1. Cryptosporidiosis, intestinal, causing diarrhoea for over 1 month
   2. *Pneumocystis carinii* pneumonia
   3. Strongyloidosis: pneumonia, CNS infection or disseminated infection*
   4. Toxoplasmosis: pneumonia or CNS infection
C.   Fungal infections
   1. Aspergillosis: CNS or disseminated infection*
   2. Candidiasis: oesophagitis
   3. Cryptococcosis: pulmonary, CNS, or disseminated infection*
D.   Bacterial infection
   1. Atypical mycobacteriosis (species other than *Mycobacterium tuberculosis* or *M. leprae*): disseminated infection*
E.   Viral infection
   1. Cytomegalovirus: pulmonary, gastrointestinal tract or CNS infection
   2. Herpes simplex virus:
      a. chronic mucocutaneous ulcers persisting more than one month, or
      b. Pulmonary, gastrointestinal tract, or disseminated infection*
   3. Progressive multifocal leukoencephalopathy ('PML' – presumed papova virus)

*Disseminated infection is involvement of lungs and multiple lymph nodes or other internal organs.

4 *The evolving epidemic*

Data coming into the CDC from investigators all over the United States showed that the incidence of AIDS was roughly doubling every six months. In September 1982, more than two cases were being diagnosed every day and by March 1983, an average of 4–5 cases per day were being reported to the CDC. The incidence of new cases from before 1981 up to the present is indicated in Figure 1.1. As of April 7 1986, a total of 19 181 cases had been reported to the CDC[5]. It is being authoritatively predicted that by 1991 a total of 270 000 people will have contracted AIDS in the United States and 179 000 will have died of it[6].

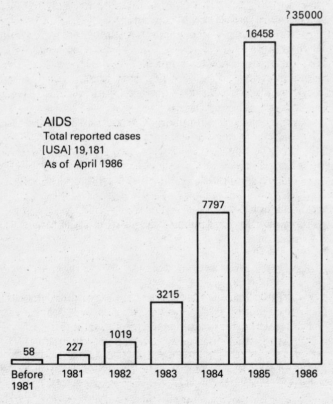

Fig. 1.1 Total reported cases of AIDS in USA pre-1981–1986

In addition to cases of fully expressed AIDS, many individuals in the same groups as those 'at risk' of developing fully expressed AIDS (e.g. gay men) were presenting for investigation or treatment with a lesser form of AIDS, which came to be referred to as the AIDS-Related Complex (ARC). Individuals with ARC frequently had a combination of various indicators of ill-health without having frank opportunistic infections or other conditions described in the surveillance definition of AIDS. Frequently they presented with unexplained, persistent and generalized swollen lymph glands (this by itself became known as either 'persistent, generalized lymphadenopathy' – PGL, or the 'lymphadenopathy syndrome' – LAS), almost always including cervical and axillary lymphy nodes[7]. In addition, individuals with ARC frequently complained of fever, profuse night sweats, fatigue and weight loss. All these patients showed abnormalities in tests for cell-mediated immunity. Some individuals with ARC progress to fully expressed AIDS. Many do not[8]. ARC is discussed in detail in Chapter 5.

For every case of AIDS, there would be ten cases of ARC. The numbers started to look astronomical.

Towards the end of 1981, the first patient diagnosed as suffering from AIDS was seen in a London hospital[9] – AIDS had arrived in the United Kingdom.

Data released from the Communicable Disease Surveillance Centre (CDSC) at Colindale reflected a similar pattern of spread to that seen in the United States. Indeed, the growth of new cases reflected the American pattern; it was merely three years behind. The number of UK cases is reflected in Figure 1.2. As of September 26, 1986, a total of 512 cases of fully expressed AIDS had been reported to the CDSC[10].

Most individuals contracting AIDS are men (Figure 1.3), and are in the age range 20–49 years, the median age being 34 (Figure 1.4).

'At risk' groups

Although in both the United States and the United Kingdom AIDS was first recognised in young, male homosexuals, it became clear from the early months of the epidemic that AIDS was not confined to either group. Most individuals in whom AIDS has been diagnosed are men with either homosexual or bisexual life styles. Also at risk are intravenous substance abusers, persons with haemophilia, the heterosexual sex partners of persons with AIDS or at risk for AIDS, recipients of transfused blood or blood components, or children from families in which one or both parents had AIDS or were in one of the 'at risk'

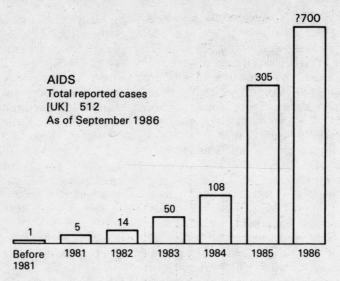

Fig. 1.2   Total reported cases of AIDS in UK pre-1981–1986

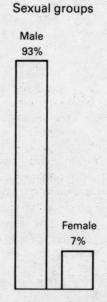

Fig. 1.3   Incidence of cases of AIDS according to sex

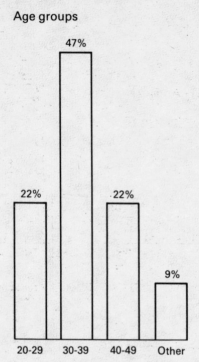

Fig. 1.4 Incidence of cases of AIDS according to age

groups for developing AIDS[11]. Figure 1.5 shows the collated average percentage breakdown of the different groups of individuals who have developed AIDS in the United States and in the United Kingdom.

Although currently most cases in the UK are associated with gay men, recent reports from Edinburgh suggest that as many as 85 per cent of individuals in that city who abuse intravenous drugs may now be infected with the agent which causes AIDS[12]. There is every reason to suspect that intravenous substance abusers will make up a significant number of UK cases of AIDS within the next year or two.

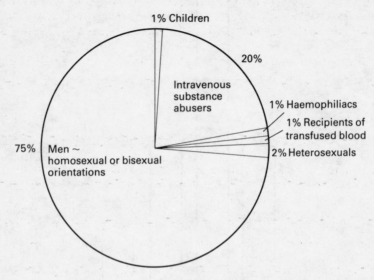

Fig. 1.5 Collated average percentage breakdown of groups of individuals who have developed AIDS in the USA and UK

Groupings of individuals at risk of developing AIDS vary in different parts of the world. In Central Africa, homosexuals do not make up a significant number of people with AIDS. There, the major 'at risk' group is all sexually active individuals, especially in towns and cities, and especially those who lead a sexually promiscuous life style[13].

Although the major 'at risk' groups have remained relatively constant in the USA and UK, it is more than likely that there will be substantial drifting into the heterosexual population. This is because we now understand the means of disease acquisition and some individuals in the current 'at risk' groups, e.g. bisexual men, intravenous substance abusers and prostitutes, are acting as a 'bridging group,' carrying the infection into sections of the population who have so far escaped infection[14].

AIDS in Europe

The first European cases were seen, it is now realized, before 1979, in France and West Germany and by the beginning of 1986, nearly 2000 cases throughout Europe had been reported to the World Health

Organization Collaborating Centre[15]. AIDS was to be seen in every country in Western Europe and, by 1986, reports of AIDS in Eastern European countries were being published[16]. In general, the same 'at risk' groups were seen in European cases, with one exception. That was the experience in France and Belgium, where there was a relatively high incidence related to the 'African connection.' Many of the cases reported in these two countries were African immigrants from the upper Congo basin or European visitors to that area, principally Zaire, Uganda, Chad and Ghana.

Mortality

AIDS is a condition associated with an extremely high case fatality rate. The overall mortality rate is 40 per cent, rising to 86 per cent for those patients diagnosed early in the epidemic. It is likely that mortality in cases reported more than two years ago will approach 100 per cent. The individual prognosis in people with AIDS varies according to their presenting illnesses. For patients with opportunistic infection, such as pneumocystosis, the average survival time is approximately eight months – none surviving more than 24 months from the date of diagnosis of the first episode.

For patients with Kaposi's sarcoma, without concurrent opportunistic infection, the average survival time is approximately 16 months, with perhaps 25 per cent surviving beyond 24 months. However, the prognosis in Kaposi's sarcoma is related to the staging classification of the disease.

In general, slightly more than half of all patients with AIDS will die within 18 months of diagnosis and, by 36 months from date of diagnosis, 80 per cent will be dead[17, 18].

Revision of the case definition of AIDS

The definition of AIDS outlined by the CDC in 1982 has been extremely useful as it is precise, consistently interpreted, and highly specific. However since the introduction of blood tests in 1985 which can detect whether or not an individual has been exposed to the AIDS virus (formerly known as HTLV-III/LAV), in May 1986 the official name for this virus was termed 'the Human Immunodeficiency Viruses, or HIV'. HIV will be used in this text to refer to the aetiological agent of AIDS; the CDC developed a more inclusive definition and classification of AIDS for diagnosis, treatment, and prevention, as well as for epidemiological studies and special surveys. The following refinements (Table 1.2) were adopted in the case definition of AIDS.

Table 1.2   AIDS — Revision of case definition — 1985[19]

1. In the absence of opportunistic diseases required by the current case definition, any of the following diseases will be considered indicative of AIDS if the patient has a positive serologic or virologic test for HTLV-III/LAV:

    (1) disseminated histoplasmosis (not confined to lungs or lymph nodes), diagnosed by culture, histology, or antigen detection;
    (2) isosporiasis, causing chronic diarrhoea (over 1 month), diagnosed by histology or stool microscopy;
    (3) bronchial or pulmonary candidiasis, diagnosed by microscopy or by presence of characteristic white plaques grossly on the bronchial mucosa (not by culture alone);
    (4) non-Hodgkin's lymphoma of high-grade pathologic type (diffuse, undifferentiated) and of B-cell or unknown immunologic phenotype, diagnosed by biopsy;
    (5) histologically confirmed Kaposi's sarcoma in patients who are 60 years old or older when diagnosed.

2. In the absence of the opportunistic diseases required by the current case definition, a histologically confirmed diagnosis of chronic lymphoid interstitial pneumonitis in a child (under 13 years of age) will be considered indicative of AIDS unless test(s) for HTLV-III/LAV are negative.

3. Patients who have a lymphoreticular malignancy diagnosed more than 3 months after the diagnosis of an opportunistic disease used as a marker for AIDS will no longer be excluded as AIDS cases.

4. To increase the specificity of the case definition, patients will be excluded as AIDS cases if they have a negative result on testing for serum antibody to HTLV-III/LAV, have no other type of HTLV-III/LAV test with a positive result, and do not have a low number of T-helper lymphocytes or a low ratio of T-helper to T-suppressor lymphocytes. In the absence of test results, patients satisfying all other criteria in the definition will continue to be included.

References

1. CDC (1981). Pneumocystis pneumonia. Los Angeles. *MMWR*, 30(21): 250-2
2. CDC (1981). Kaposi's sarcoma and Pneumocystis pneumonia among homosexual men. New York City and California. *MMWR*, 30(25): 305-8.
3. CDC (1981). Follow-up on Kaposi's sarcoma and Pneumocystis pneumonia. *MMWR*, 30(33):409-10
4. CDC (1982). Update on acquired immune deficiency (AIDS). United States. *MMWR*, 31:507-14
5. Public Health Laboratory Service. (1986). HTLV 3 Antibody Reports: Weeks 86/14-17. *CDR* 86/17
6. Barnes, D.M. (1986). Grim projections for AIDS epidemic. *Science*, June 27, 232(4758):1589-90
7. CDC (1982). Persistent, generalized lymphadenopathy among homosexual males. *MMWR*, 31(19):249-51
8. Mathur-Wagh, U., *et al* (1984). Longitudinal study of persistent generalised lymphadenopathy in homosexual men; relation to acquired immunodeficiency syndrome. *Lancet*, May 12, i(8385):1033-38
9. DuBois, R.M., *et al* (1981). Primary *Pneumocystis carinii* and cytomegalovirus infections. *Lancet*. December 12, ii(8259):1339
10. Public Health Laboratory Service, *CDR* 26 September, 1986, 86/39: 3-4.
11. CDC (1986) update: Acquired Immunodeficiency Syndrome. United States, *MMWR*, 35(2):17-21
12. Robertson, J.R., *et al* (1986). Epidemic of AIDS related virus (HTLV-III/LAV) infection among intravenous drug abusers. *British Medical Journal*, February 22, 292:527-30
13. Anonymous (1985). AIDS: the search for clues. *WHO Chronicle*, 39(6):207-11
14. Anonymous (1985). AIDS: where do we go from here? *WHO Chronicle*, 39(3):98-103
15. Daniels, V.G. (1985). *AIDS, The Acquired Immune Deficiency Syndrome*. MTP Press Ltd. London, pp 3-4
16. *IME Bulletin*. October 1985. London, p 11
17. DeVita, V.T. Jr. *et al* (1985). *AIDS — Etiology, Diagnosis, Treatment and Prevention*. J.B. Lippincott Co. Philadelphia, pp 6-7
18. Daniels (1985). *op. cit.*, p 88
19. CDC (1985). Revision of the case definition of Acquired Immunodeficiency Syndrome for national reporting. United States, *MMWR*, 34(25):373-5

2

AIDS – The Cause

From the beginning of the epidemic, AIDS exhibited all the classic signs of an infectious disease and the only convincing explanation for its cause was the emergence of a new infectious agent. An infective aetiology was consistent with the geographical clustering of early cases and epidemiological proof of case-to-case contact[1,2], the newness of the disease, the pattern of groups at risk, its occurrence, within the same time scale, in the diverse groups affected, and finally, its exponential spread. Various researchers independently discovered the causative agent of AIDS at approximately the same time and named the virus responsible: LAV – the lymphadenopathy-associated virus[3], HTLV-III – Human T cell leukemia (lymphotropic) virus type III[4], and ARV – AIDS-associated retrovirus[5]. In May 1986 a subcommittee of the International Committee on the Taxonomy of Viruses proposed that the AIDS retroviruses be officially designated as the 'human immuno-deficiency viruses' (HIV). Although in the UK, HTLV-III has generally been used to refer to the aetiological agent of AIDS, it is likely that in the future, HIV will become the accepted name for this agent, and thus will be used in this text.

Characteristics of HIV

Viruses are composed of a core of **nucleic acid** (either deoxyribonucleic acid – DNA, or ribonucleic acid – RNA) which constitute the viral **genome** (genetic composition). The genome is enclosed within and intimately attached to a protein outer shell, known as the **capsid**. The capsid is built from numerous small units (capsomeres) and the capsid and genome are closely integrated to form a **nucleocapsid** of an exactly defined symmetry. The capsids of different viruses have different shapes (symmetry). Some are cubical (icosahedral), others helical, and still others are so complex that their symmetry has not yet been described. The capsid serves to protect the delicate nucleic acid. The proteins of the capsid have a special affinity for specific receptor sites on host cells, which allow the virus to attach itself to and invade this cell, initiating the process of infection (Figure 2.1).

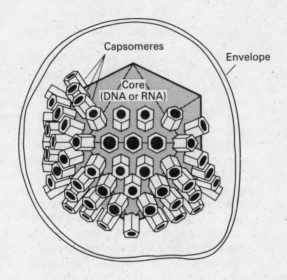

Fig. 2.1 The structure of a virus (with acknowledgement to *Medical Microbiology*, Volume I, published by Churchill Livingstone)

Viruses can exist outside cells (extracellular forms), the complete infective viral particle (the genome in the core surrounded by the capsid) being known as a **virion**. Some virions are enclosed in a lipoprotein **envelope**, derived from material (nuclear and cytoplasmic membranes) in the cells they infect, which clings to them when they escape, by the process of budding. Viruses are not classified as true cells as they do not contain a limiting plasma membrane, cytoplasm, ribosomes, mitochondria, enzymes to generate high energy bonds, or muramic acid in their outer coverings. However, because they contain nucleic acid, the fundamental property of life, they are able to reproduce, but *only inside a cell*, thus being intracellular parasites. Because of this fundamental feature of viruses, they have often been described as 'genetic material in search of a living cell, in which to reproduce.'

When a virion enters a cell (the **host cell**), it loses its protein capsid (and lipoprotein envelope, if it has one). The viral nucleic acid takes over the genetic material of the host cell, along with the cell's raw materials, energy-producing and metabolic systems. It then commands the host cell to produce more viruses; several hundred new viruses can be produced in each infected host cell which then go on to infect other cells.

Virions are extremely small, varying in diameter from 18 to 300 nanometre (a nanometre, or 'nm,' is one-thousandth part of a micrometre or one-millionth part of a millimetre). There are hundreds of viruses which can infect man. They are usually classified in groups depending on the composition of their nucleic acid, i.e., either DNA viruses or RNA viruses.

HIV is a special type of virus known as a **retrovirus**. Retroviruses are RNA viruses which have a lipid-containing membrane surrounding the capsid. Retroviruses also have a special viral enzyme, known as **reverse transcriptase**, which allows the virus to make a DNA copy of its RNA genetic material, facilitating its integration into the genetic material of the host cell. Once inserted into the genetic material of the host cell, it directs this cell to produce more RNA retroviruses. Reverse transcriptase refers to the process of making DNA from RNA, the presence of this enzyme being a unique feature of all retroviruses. Although retroviruses were known to cause disease in some animals (leukaemia in cats), it was not thought that they were involved in human disease. In 1978, a new retrovirus, associated with the aetiology of an aggressive, human, adult T-cell leukemia and named '**Human T cell Leukemia virus**' (HTLV), was isolated by Robert Gallo[6]. In 1982, Gallo identified another similar, but distinct retrovirus from a patient with hairy cell leukaemia. This was named '**Human T cell Leukemia virus, type II**' (HTLV-II)[7]. **Human T cell Leukemia viruses** (HTLV) were especially (but not exclusively) attracted to T lymphocytes of the helper subgroup, which became their targets. This attraction, or 'tropism' for helper cells, made them a likely candidate for investigation into the aetiology of AIDS as it was known that patients with this disease had a decreased number of helper cells. The possibility that a retrovirus of the HTLV group was involved in the aetiology of AIDS was first reported by Robert Gallo in February 1982[8]. This was followed by Luc Montagnier's discovery of the **lymphadenopathy-associated virus** (LAV) in 1983, and Gallo's discovery of the new type of **human T cell leukemia virus**, type III (HTLV-III). In 1984, Dr. Jay Levy in San Francisco also identified the AIDS virus, which he named the **AIDS-associated retrovirus** (ARV). It is now clear that all of these viruses are different isolates of the same virus.

Pathophysiology of infection with HIV

HIV has a special affinity for helper cells and infects some but certainly not all of them. Those infected are turned into virus-producing cells and eventually destroyed. Viral replication increases when the infected T-helper cell is activated. Helper cells can be activated by infections (e.g. sexually transmitted diseases) or by the presence of substances containing non-infective antigens such as the antigenic components of semen or concentrated Factor VIII. Newly produced viruses are liberated by 'budding' out from the host cell and infect more helper cells, eventually leading to their destruction. The presence of HIV in some helper cells may also provoke an autoimmune response against non-infected helper cells, causing further destruction of these important cells[9].

Once helper cells are depleted, B lymphocytes are inefficient as they require the 'help' of helper cells to produce specific antibody. Cytotoxic T-cell and lymphokine-producing T-cell activity is also impaired, resulting in a decreased ability of the immune system to destroy neoplastic and virus infected cells. Some macrophages, which also have special receptors, similar to those found on helper cells (T4 antigens) may be directly infected by HIV.

A sinister feature of HIV infection is recent evidence that some cells in the brain (glial cells) are also directly infected[10], causing encephalopathy in patients with AIDS. More ominously, the fact that HIV can infect and slowly replicate within brain cells suggest that this retrovirus belongs to a subfamily known as '**lentiviruses**.' An infamous member of this subfamily is the '**visna virus**' which causes a slowly progressive central nervous system deterioration in sheep. The chilling suggestion is that HIV may cause neurological disease (e.g. dementia) in individuals infected, who are currently asymptomatic[11, 12]. Considering the vast numbers of individuals who are now infected and the continuing growth of infection in the community, the possibility of significant numbers of individuals escaping fully expressed AIDS, but eventually succumbing to neurological consequences of infection, leaves little doubt as to the seriousness of this epidemic.

Co-factors

Once infected with HIV, ultimate disease expression may depend on the presence of one or more additional factors (co-factors). The presence of these various co-factors may explain why some individuals infected with HIV succumb to AIDS, or AIDS-related complex (ARC), while others remain asymptomatic. Co-factors currently being investigated include:

A genetic predisposition to disease expression.   The degree of susceptibility to HIV may be related to a genetically determined immune response controlled by an individual's major histocompatibility complex (MHC). The MHC is a system of genetically linked antigens (termed human leucocyte antigens group A, or 'HLA') controlled by a complex of genes on the 6th chromosome. These genes occur on four different regions (loci) of this chromosome, loci A, B, C and D. The exact arrangement of these genes differs in different individuals. Those located on locus D (HLA-D) are of special importance as they have been associated with a predisposition to certain immunological diseases (principally, autoimmune disorders). There is an increased incidence of Kaposi's sarcoma in individuals with AIDS, who have a special HLA-D antigen known as HLA-DR5, and who do not possess another HLA-D antigen, known as HLA-DR3 (i.e., they are HLA-DR5 positive and HLA-DR3 negative)[13, 14]. This finding suggests that a genetic predisposition may be one aspect that determines final disease expression in individuals infected with HIV.

The presence of other latent viral infections.   Many individuals in the community are infected with different types of **herpesviruses**. These enveloped DNA viruses include: **herpes simplex virus** (types 1 & 2), **Varicella-zoster virus, cytomegalovirus (CMV)**, and the **Epstein-Barr virus** (EBV). Although these viruses can cause overt disease, in most individuals they cause latent (but persistent) infection, frequently with no signs or symptoms. Once infected, the viruses lie dormant, but can be reactivated occasionally, causing recurrent disease.

CMV.   CMV infection is common in the community and approximately 50 per cent of women of childbearing age have CMV antibody, which reflects persistent infection[15]. This virus is found in and shed from urine, semen, and saliva. Both primary and recurrent infections are generally asymptomatic. Most sexually active homosexual men have serological evidence of persistent infection[16]. CMV infection in immunocompromised individuals increases their susceptibility to opportunistic infections[17] and can cause various immunological abnormalities[18], [19]. All patients with AIDS, ARC and Kaposi's sarcoma are CMV seropositive[20, 21].

EBV.   EBV infection, like other **herpesviruses**, causes a persistent carrier state, following primary infection. This virus, found in saliva, has a particular affinity for B lymphocytes, which have special receptors allowing EBV to infect them. Primary infection may cause infectious mononucleosis. EBV is also associated with the causation of a malignant lymphoma (Burkitt's lymphoma) and B Cell lymphomas in patients with AIDS[22]. All patients with AIDS have serological evidence of EBV infection[23].

Herpes simplex virus (HSV). In general, infection with HSV type 1 causes herpes labialis (lesions on the lips) and keratitis and HSV type 2 causes genital herpes. A large proportion of homosexual men (90–100%) have serological evidence of infection with HSV type 2[24] and while in many of these individuals latent infection is asymptomatic, some have recurrent genital and perirectal lesions. Primary disease and reactivation of HSV type 2 disease is commonly seen in AIDS[25].

Varicella-zoster virus. This virus causes chickenpox (varicella) and shingles (zoster). Reactivation of the virus (acquired originally perhaps in childhood varicella infection) is commonly seen in the AIDS-related complex (especially in PGL).

Other possible co-factors. During anal intercourse, semen can be absorbed from the rectal mucosa and repeated exposure to allogeneic sperm may induce immunosuppression[26, 27]. Defects in helper to suppressor cell ratios similar to those seen in AIDS have been reported in men who engaged in receptive anal intercourse[28].

The origins of the virus

It may be that the exact origins of AIDS will never be completely elicited. There are, however, certain facts that have led to a more or less general agreement as to the source of this epidemic. It is plausible to conclude that HIV is a pathogen new to the human race, probably resulting from a non-pathogenic primate retrovirus, which made a 'species jump' from the African green monkey to humans. There is widespread evidence that green monkeys in Africa have been infected with a virus similar to HIV for many years[29], although it does not cause disease in these animals. This virus is referred to as **Simian T-lymphotropic virus type III** – STLV-III (AGM). This retrovirus is most likely the progenitor agent from which HIV either mutated or recombined into the human population. The virus may have been transferred to humans as a result of an animal bite, or by humans eating the uncooked meat (especially brains) of these monkeys. Cases of AIDS in Africa became known at about the same time (1981) as American and European cases, although it is likely that human HIV infection existed in Africa long before the disease was recognised. AIDS is now epidemic in some central and east African countries (Zambia, Zaire, Rwanda, Uganda, and parts of Tanzania). The current pandemic may have started in Africa and have spread simultaneously to the USA, Haiti and

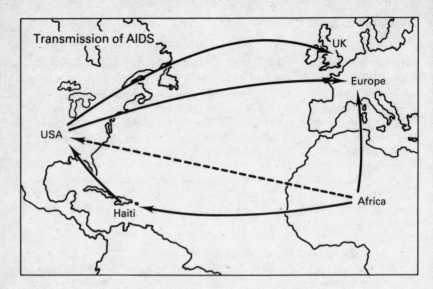

Fig. 2.2   The spread of HIV

Europe. Certainly many Haitians lived in Zaire from the early 1960s to
the middle 1970s, and then moved to the United States, Europe, or
returned to Haiti. It is likely that the spread of AIDS into the UK
occurred via British tourists returning from American holidays. However the spread of AIDS into the rest of Europe was more likely a direct
result of African links (Figure 2.2).

Other retroviruses, similar to both STLV-III (AGM) and HTLV-III,
have recently been identified. Luc Montagnier has identified a retrovirus (LAV-II) from patients with AIDS which is significantly different
from HTLV-III (LAV-I) and Max Essex has discovered a human retrovirus which infects T-cells, but does not destroy them. This retrovirus is
more like STLV-III (AGM) than like HTLV-III, and has been termed
HTLV-IV[30]. There is most likely a continuum of retroviruses involved,
from STLV-III (AGM) to HTLV-IV and LAV-II, which have developed, and show variations in their characteristics. HIV itself shows
marked 'antigenic drift,' i.e. it is capable of changing its antigenic proteins and producing new 'strains,' much like the influenza virus.
Intense research is continuing into the origins of the putative progenitor
virus of this disease, as new information may lead to a more effective
treatment strategy and could lead to the development of an effective
vaccine.

Incubation period

AIDS is associated with a long incubation period. In some individuals, exposure to HIV is initially followed by an acute, febrile, glandular fever type of illness, lasting 3 to 14 days, during which patients presents with complaints of fever and night sweats, general malaise and lethargy, myalgia and arthralgia. Many patients with this acute HIV infection also complain of lymphadenopathy, sore throat, anorexia, nausea and vomiting, headaches and photophobia, diarrhoea, and a roseola-like rash[31, 32]. This acute illness is a direct result of initial HIV infection or, in some individuals, due to a reactivation of **cytomegalo-virus** (CMV) infection secondary to a moderate immunosuppression caused by HIV infection[33]. The acute reaction to HIV infection, which does not occur in all infected individuals, may precede or follow the developments of antibodies (seroconversion) to HIV. Antibodies to HIV (anti-HIV) are generally produced within three to six months. These antibodies are non-neutralizing antibodies of the IgG class.

Important points for nurses to note regarding seroconversion are: (1) some individuals infected with HIV fail to produce anti-bodies[34, 35, 36]; (2) during the lag period between exposure and seroconversion individuals are able to transmit infection, and may, in fact, be highly infectious during this phase; (3) a decline in detectable antibody levels is sometimes seen in patients with advanced, clinical AIDS[37]. Therefore, from a nursing point of view, a negative blood test for anti-HIV does not necessarily imply that a patient has not been infected with this virus. Following seroconversion, there is usually a long latent period (up to five years or longer) before some individuals develop either AIDS or manifestations of ill health due to HIV infection.

By this time, twenty per cent of individuals infected with HIV will have developed fully expressed AIDS, a further thirty per cent will have developed signs and symptoms of the AIDS-related complex (ARC), and the remaining fifty per cent will have remained asymptomatic[38]. Whether or not they will remain asymptomatic in the years to come is not presently known. It is presumed, however, that they will remain infectious.

References

1. Auerbach, D.M., Bennett, J.V., Brachman, P.J. & the CDC Task Force. (1982). Epidemiologic aspects of the current outbreak of Kaposi's sarcoma and opportunistic infections. *New England Journal of Medicine* (January 26) 306(4):248–52

2. Gazzard, B.G., Farthing, C., *et al*. (1984). Clinical findings and serological evidence of HTLV-III infections in homosexual contacts of patients with AIDS and Persistent Generalised Lymphadenopathy. *Lancet*. (September 1) ii(8401):480–83

3. Barre-Sinoussi, F., Chermann, J.C., *et al*. (1983). Isolation of a T-lymphotropic retrovirus from a patient at risk for acquired immune deficiency syndrome (AIDS). *Science* (May 20) 220(4599):868–71

4. Gallo, R.C., Salahuddin, S.Z., *et al*. (1984). Frequent detection and isolation of cytopathic retroviruses (HTLV-III) from patients with AIDS and at risk for AIDS. *Science* (May 4) 224(4648):500–3

5. Levy, J.A., Hoffman, A.D., *et al*. (1984). Isolation of lymphocytopathic retroviruses from San Francisco patients with AIDS. *Science* 225:840

6. Poiesz, B.J., Ruscetti, F.W., *et al*. (1980). Detection and isolation of type-C retrovirus particles from fresh and cultured lymphocytes of a patient with cutaneous T-cell lymphoma. *Proceedings of the National Academy of Science*. (USA). 77:7415–19

7. Kalyanaraman, V.S., Sarngaddharan, M.G., *et al*. (1982). A new subtype of human T-cell leukemia virus (HTLV-II) associated with a T-cell variant of hairy cell leukemia. *Science* 218:571–73

8. Gallo, R.C., Essex, M., Gross, L. (1982). Human T-cell leukemia/lymphoma virus. Cold Spring Harbor Press, New York, 1984

9. Montagnier, L. (1986). Lymphadenopathy Associated Virus: its role in the pathogenesis of AIDS and related diseases. Acquired Immunodeficiency Syndrome, edited by E. Klien, *Progress in Allergy*, Vol. 37, pp. 46–64. Karger. Basel. 1986

10. Levy, J.A., Hollander, H., *et al*. (1985). Isolation of AIDS-associated retroviruses from cerebrospinal fluid and brain of patients with neurological symptoms. *Lancet*. September 14: ii(8455):568–8

11. Maddox, J. (1986). Further anxieties about AIDS. *Nature* (January 2) 319:9

12. Seale, J. (1985). AIDS virus infection: prognosis and transmission. *Journal of the Royal Society of Medicine*. August 78:613–5

13. Friedman-Kien, A.E., Laubenstein, L.J., and Rubenstein, P., *et al*. (1982). Disseminated Kaposi's sarcoma in homosexual men. *Annals of Internal Medicine*, 96:693

14. Giraldo, G., and Berth, E. (1986). The involvement of Cytomegalovirus in Acquired Immune Deficiency Syndrome and Kaposi's sarcoma, *in Acquired Immunodeficiency Syndrome*, ed. by E. Klien (*Progress in Allergy* Vol. 37) p 325

15. Peckham, C. and Jeffries, D. (1986). Cytomegalovirus and the pregnant woman. (February) Draft Information paper on CMV prepared for and endorsed by the Advisory Committee on Dangerous Pathogens (ACDP). DHSS. London

16. Drew, W.L., Mintz, L., Miner, R.C., *et al*. (1981). Presence of cytomegalovirus in homosexual men. *Journal of Infectious Diseases*. (February) 143(2) 188–92

17. Rand, K.H., Pollard, R.B., and Merigan, T.C. (1978). Increased pulmonary superinfection in cardiac-transplant patients undergoing primary

cytomegalovirus infection. *New England Journal of Medicine*. (April 27). 298(17) 951–53

18. Hirsch, M.S. (1984). *Cytomegalovirus-leukocyte interactions*: *in* Plotkin, Michelson, Pagano, Rapp. *CMV: Pathogenesis and prevention of human infections. Births defects* (Vol. 20), 161–73 (Liss, New York)

19. Carney, W.P., Rubin, R.H., *et al.* (1981). T-lymphocyte subsets in cyto-megalovirus mononucleosis. *Journal of Immunology*. (June) 126(6) 2114–16

20. Drew, W.L., Constant, M.A., Miner, R.C., Huang, E.S., Ziegler, J.L., *et al.* (1982). Cytomegalovirus and Kaposi's sarcoma in young homo-sexual men. *Lancet*. (July 17) ii(8290):125–7

21. Quinnan, G.V., Jr., Mazur, H., Rook, A.H., *et al.* (1984). Herpes infec-tions in the acquired immune deficiency syndrome. *Journal of the Amer-ican Medical Association*. 252:72–77

22. Ernberg I. (1986). The role of Epstein-Barr Virus in lymphomas of homo-sexual males, in *Acquired Immunodeficiency Syndrome*, ed. by E. Klein (*Progress in Allergy* Vol. 37) *op. cit.*

23. Rogers, M.F., Morens, O.M., Stewart, J.A., *et al.* (1983). National case-control study of Kaposi's sarcoma and *Pneumocystis carinii* pneumonia in homosexual men: Part 2, Laboratory results. *Annals of Internal Medicine*. (August) 99(2) 151–8

24. Ibid.

25. Siegal, F.P., Lopez, C., Hammer, G.S., *et al.* (1981). Severe acquired immunodeficiency in male homosexuals manifested by chronic perianal ulcerative herpes simplex lesions. *New England Journal of Medicine*. (December 10) 305(24):1439–44

26. Shearer, G. (1983). AIDS: A consequence of allogeneic Ia-antigen recog-nition. *Immunology Today*. (July) 4(7) 181 & 184–5

27. Witkin, S.S., Sonnabend, J., Richards, J.M. & Purtilo, D.T. (1983). Induction of antibody to asialo GMl by spermatozoa and its occurrence in the sera of homosexual men with the acquired immune deficiency syndrome (AIDS). *Clinical and Experimental Immunology*. (November) 54(2) 346–50

28. Mavligit, G.M., Talpaz, M., Hsia, F.T., *et al.* (1984). Chronic immune stimulation by sperm alloantigens. Support for the hypothesis that spermatozoa induce immune dysregulation in homosexual males. *Journal of the American Medical Association*. (January 13) 251(2) 237–41

29. Biggar, R.J., (1986). The AIDS problem in Africa. *Lancet*. (January 11) i(8472): 79–83.

30. Walgate, R. and Palca, J. (1986). AIDS Research. *Nature*. (April 3) Vol. 320:385

31. Cooper, D.A., Gold, J., Maclean, P., *et al.* (1985). Acute AIDS Retro-virus Infection – definition of a clinical illness associated with serocon-version. *Lancet*. (March 9) i(8428):537–40

32. Lindskov, R., Orskov Lindhardt, B., Weismann, K., *et al.* (1986). Acute HTLV-III Infection with roseola-like rash. *Lancet*. (February 22) i(8478):447

33. Farthing, C. and Gazzard, B. (1985). Acute illness associated with HTLV-III seroconversion. *Lancet*. (April 20) i(8434):935–6

34. Mayer, K.H., Stoddard, A.M., McCusker, J., *et al.* (1986). Human T-Lymphotropic Virus Type III in high-risk, antibody-negative homosexual men. *Annals of Internal Medicine.* (February) 104:194–6
35. Salahuddin, S.Z., Markham, P.D., Redfield, R.R., *et al.* (1984). HTLV-III in symptom-free seronegative persons. *Lancet.* (December 22/29) ii(8417/8):1418–20
36. Groopman, J.E., Hartzband, P.I., Shulman, L., *et al.* (1985). Antibody seronegative human T-lymphotropic virus type III (HTLV-III)-infected patients with acquired immunodeficiency syndrome or related disorders. *Blood* 66:742–44
37. Levy, J.A., Kamisky, L.S., Morrow, W.J.W., *et al.* (1985). Infection by the retrovirus associated with the acquired immunodeficiency syndrome: clinical, biological, and molecular features. *Annals of Internal Medicine.* 103:694–99
38. Barnes, D.M. (1986). Grim projections for AIDS epidemic. *Science*, June 27, 232(4758):1589–90.

3

The Immunological Background to the Acquired Immune Deficiency Syndrome

An understanding of normal immune mechanisms is necessary in order to appreciate fully the immune dysfunctions seen in AIDS. Immunity, an increased resistance to infectious disease, has evolved in man over the centuries and affords essential protection, without which survival would be impossible. There are many non-specific mechanisms available to everyone, which we employ to protect ourselves against infection – non-specific in that they are used to attack all potential pathogens (microbes which cause disease). This type of immunity, referred to as **innate** immunity, is geared towards either the prevention of pathogenic invasion or containment and eventual resolution should invasion occur.

Prevention of invasion

Intact skin.   A healthy, intact skin provides a good barrier against invasion by pathogens. It is unusual, however, for skin to be perfectly intact as all of us have small or microscopic abrasions. At any rate, sweat glands, hair follicles, etc., provide an entry for many potential pathogens.

Mucous membranes and ciliated cells.   External openings of the body are guarded by mucous membranes. For example, the mouth, nose, urethra, vagina and rectum are all lined with mucous membranes. These membranes secrete sticky mucus so that when pathogens enter the body by one of these routes, many of them are impinged on these sticky, mucous surfaces. Many of these membranes are associated with cells, which have hair-like processes, known as **cilia** (e.g. the upper respiratory system) which are then able to waft pathogens away from deeper structures, eventually assisting in expelling them from the body.

pH changes.   Some areas of the body have a pH which is often hostile to many pathogens. For example, the pH of the vagina is acid and pathogens which require an alkaline medium to reproduce would not be successful in establishing infection in this environment. The pH changes in the gastro-intestinal tract, where ingested food is first mixed with saliva in an alkaline medium in the mouth, is then swallowed into the acid environment of the stomach, and eventually passed into the alkaline environment of the duodenum, can be either bacteriostatic (preventing bacterial growth) or bacteriocidal (killing bacteria) to many pathogens.

Chemical secretions. Many secretions in the body can be either bacteriocidal or -static. For example, nasal secretions, saliva, sweat and tears all contain substances known as **lysozymes**, which are bacteriocidal to many gram-positive bacteria. In the presence of **complement**, lysozymes can destroy many gram-negative bacteria. Another substance in serum is **properdin** which is also able to destroy many gram-negative bacteria and (with complement) many viruses.

Containment of invading pathogens

Effective as these non-specific mechanisms are, pathogenic invasion does occur from time to time. The body still has some fairly sophisticated, non-specific mechanisms available to deal with these pathogens, which, if successful, contain them, limit the damage and eventually destroy them. These include:

Inflammation – this is a protective mechanism, which results in an increase in local blood supply to the area under attack. This hyperaemia is the cause of the classic signs of inflammation (heat, redness, swelling and pain). With this increased blood supply come cells which are able to engage in **phagocytosis**.

Phagocytosis – the normal white blood cell count is made up of different white cells which have different functions. In every cubic millimetre of blood, there are between 8000 and 10 000 white blood cells – this is referred to as a normal **white cell count**. Making up this total white cell count are:–

(i)   Polymorphonuclear white blood cells (granulocytes).
       These account for 70 per cent of the white cells
       There are 3 different types of polymorphonuclear cells:
              – basophils – eosinophils – neutrophils
       Neutrophils account for most of the polymorphs and are actively phagocytic (basophils and eosinophils are not phagocytic cells – they have different functions)
(ii) Monocytes. These make up 5 per cent of the white cell count and these cells are also phagocytic
(iii) Lymphocytes. These make up the remaining 25 per cent of the white cell count – these cells are not phagocytic and will be

discussed later. There are two different types of lymphocytes:– **T-cells** and **B-cells**

Phagocytosis is the process by which bacteria are engulfed by neutrophils and monocytes and eventually destroyed. Other cells in the body capable of phagocytosis, are known as **macrophages**.

Other determinants of innate immunity which influence the ability of the individual to withstand infectious disease include:

Nutrition – a well nourished individual is better able to deal with an infectious process than people who are not well nourished.

Age – the very young and the very old are less able to ward off infectious diseases.

Race – some races are either more prone to or more immune from certain diseases than others.

Species – Man is immune to many of the diseases which affect animals and vice versa.

All of these factors, associated with innate immunity, offer good protection against infectious diseases. However, by themselves, they are not adequate for survival in the hostile environment in which man finds himself. We need much more specific protection and this is afforded by the specific immune response of **acquired immunity**.

Acquired immunity – the specific immune response

During the first few months of life, the infant begins to acquire protection against specific pathogens. This type of immunity, known as **acquired immunity**, allows the child to mount a specific immune response towards each pathogen the child encounters as it progresses through those first vulnerable months and years. For the first three months of its life, the child is protected by the natural, passive immunity conferred by the mother. During these first few months, antibodies from the mother pass to the child while it is still in the uterus. However, these antibodies are short-lived and by the end of three months, the child must begin to acquire its own immunity.

Acquired immunity involves two different but inter-related processes. The first process is known as **humoral immunity**.

Humoral immunity

The active agents of acquired immunity are the lymphocytes. We have already mentioned that there are two different types of lymphocytes

– the **B-lymphocytes** and the **T-lymphocytes**. Both originate from stem cells, which are manufactured in the bone marrow. Some of these stem cells, destined to become B-lymphocytes (B-cells) are known as B-cell precursors. The remaining stem cells, destined to become T-lymphocytes are, of course, T-cell precursors. The B-cell precursors migrate back to the bone marrow, where they are 'processed' into B-lymphocytes. They are known as B-lymphocytes as they were first identified in the hindgut of a bird, an area known as the 'Bursa of Fabricius.' Although humans do not have this special tissue, it is thought that they have similar areas (Bursa equivalent areas), such as the foetal liver and the bone marrow, which 'process' B-cell precursors in such a way that when they develop into fully mature B-lymphocytes, they respond in a specific manner to pathogens. The manner in which they respond is known as **humoral immunity**. B-lymphocytes account for about 30 per cent of all lymphocytes (the remaining 70 per cent being T-lymphocytes). Figure 3.1 illustrates the development of a mature B-lymphocyte.

Humoral immunity is acquired as follows: A foreign cell, be it a bacterium, a virus, a tissue cell, etc., is recognized by the body as 'not self' and referred to as an **antigen**. For the moment, we are going to think of antigens as bacteria or viruses, but they can be anything (usually a protein) which the body detects as 'different.' These antigens are 'pre-processed' by phagocytic cells (discussed later) and eventually present to the B-lymphocytes in lymphatic tissue (e.g. spleen, liver, bone marrow and lymph nodes) where the presence of this antigen stimulates the B-cell to proliferate and change into **plasma cells** and **memory cells**. Plasma cells have a specific function which is to secrete a protein substance known as **antibody**. The rate of antibody secretion is impressive, in the order of 2000 antibody molecules per second for each plasma cell. This goes on for several days until the plasma cell dies (4–5 days).

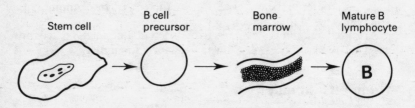

| | B cell | Bone | Mature B |
| Stem cell | precursor | marrow | lymphocyte |

Fig. 3.1　The maturation of a B-lymphocyte

The antibody then combines with antigen. This combination of anti-body plus antigen equals an **immune complex**. Antibodies protect the individual in several ways; firstly, the antibody attacks the antigen's cell wall, weakening and eventually destroying it; this is known as lysis.

More importantly, when the antibody 'coats' or attaches itself to an antigen, the formation of immune complexes sets off a cascade of chemical events in which certain enzymes in the blood (complement enzymes) become activated in a sequential manner, resulting in active **complement**. Complement has two important functions: it initiates a local inflammatory reaction at the invasion site, which increases the local blood supply, and secondly, by-products of inflammation chemi-cally attract neutrophils, monocytes and other phagocytic cells known as **macrophages** (discussed later) to the area under attack. This chemical attraction of phagocytic cells to the invasion site is known as **chemotaxis**. Some antigens are destroyed by direct cell wall damage when coated by complement.

We can see that it is critically important for plasma cells to secrete antibody. There are two important points to remember: the antibody produced is specific to that particular antigen, e.g. if the antigen was the chickenpox virus, then the antibody produced would bind only to the chickenpox virus – it would not bind to the measles virus. Secondly, antibody is formed in a sequential manner, something like: antibody 1, antibody 2, antibody 3, etc. Hence, soon after invasion, antibody 1 is formed, then in a week or so, antibody 2 is formed, etc. If we took a sample of blood at week two of the infection, we might find the first antibody still there, but disappearing, and the 2nd antibody just appearing. Perhaps antibody 1 would disappear within a month but antibody 3 would stay in the serum for years, or for life. This would be important, as the presence of antibody 1 would be a diagnostic marker of acute infection while antibody 3 would be a marker of previous expo-sure. However, all the antibodies would be antibodies to that specific antigen (e.g. the chickenpox virus) – they would simply be different classes of the antibody.

All the different classes of antibodies are collectively known as **immunoglobulins**. They are not of course called antibody 1, antibody 2, etc., but rather IgM, IgG, IgA, IgD and IgE (the 'Ig' stands for **immunoglobulin** – hence, the classes of immunoglobulin are M, G, A, D, and E). A few points about the different classes of immuno-globulins:

IgM – this important class of antibody usually appears early in the course of an infectious disease and disappears as the patient recovers. Hence it is a marker of acute infection. It accounts for about 6 per cent of the total amount of immunoglobulin formed working by neutralizing pathogens (especially viruses) by lysis or by enhancing phagocytosis.

IgG (Gamma Globulin) – this class of antibody accounts for 70–90 per cent of all the immunoglobulin formed, being especially useful at activating complement and promoting phagocytosis. It remains in the body for long periods of time (years, or a lifetime) hence its presence is not an indication of acute infection, but rather of previous exposure.

IgA – accounts for up to 13 per cent of the total amount of immunoglobulin formed, but accounts for over 90 per cent of the immunoglobulin found on mucosal surfaces (e.g. nose, mouth, etc.) and protects the body by neutralizing antigens that enter by these routes.

IgD – accounts for about 18 per cent of the total amount of immunoglobulin formed – not much is known for certain about its specific function.

IgE – only accounts for about 0.002 per cent of immunoglobulin formed and this can bind to 'mast cells' causing these cells to release vasoactive substances, such as histamine and serotonin, which are responsible for the common signs and symptoms of acute allergic reactions.

Memory cells – when provoked by the presence of an antigen, both T-cells and B-cells produce *memory cells*, clones of the stimulated parent cell. Should the individual encounter the same antigen any time in the future, the cascade of events which constitute a specific immune response will be accelerated. This is because memory cells 'remember' the specific antigen and respond quickly.

Mast cells – these are special cells, which are capable of releasing substances such as heparin, histamine, serotonin and SRS (slow-reacting-substance) of anaphylaxis when stimulated to do so by IgE immunoglobulin bound to their surface. One type of polymorphonuclear white blood cell, a basophil, is a type of circulating mast cell – others are 'fixed' in most tissues of the body, e.g. lung tissue.

Summary   Humoral immunity is the process whereby B-lymphocytes, provoked by the presence of an antigen, proliferate and undergo change, some changing into memory cells, but most changing into plasma cells. Plasma cells have just one function – to secrete specific antibody which can combine with the antigen, forming immune complexes, activating the complement system and by different methods, eventually destroying the invading pathogen.

Cell-mediated immunity

The other process involved in acquired immunity is that of **cell-mediated immunity**. This involves the **T-lymphocytes** which are derived from the same stem cells as B-lymphocytes, but which migrate to the **thymus gland** for processing, rather than to bone marrow and other bursa equivalent areas. In the thymus gland, these T-cell precursors are 'processed' to react differently when they encounter antigens. Mature T-lymphocytes account for about 70 per cent of the total number of lymphocytes. When they encounter an antigen, they differentiate into several different sub-sets:

Lymphokine producing cells (T-D cells) – these cells release various **lymphokines**, substances which mediate other inflammatory cells and phagocytic cells. Several lymphokines are released by T-D cells, including **interferon** and **interleukin 2**. Interferon has a direct anti-virus effect but also activates a cell, known as a **Natural Killer cell** – (NK cell). These cells, once activated, are involved in preventing the development of tumours in the body. If they were defective, there would be an increased incidence of cancer in an individual. Other lymphokines act on other cells, enhancing inflammation and chemotaxis.

Cytotoxic cells (T-C cells) – these important cells are necessary to destroy cells harbouring viruses. They require T-helper cells to activate and any deficiency in cytotoxic cell activity would render the individual at increased risk of viral infections.

Regulator cells – these cells regulate the activity of all the other sub-sets of both B-cells, and T-cells. There are two different regulator cells: **helper cells** which 'help' plasma cells effectively secrete specific antibody, 'help' cytotoxic cells activate, and 'help' lymphokine-producing cells activate and release their various chemical mediators. **Suppressor cells** will eventually 'suppress' helper cells, cytotoxic and lymphokine-producing cells when the emergency is over. Helper cells are also known as T4 lymphocytes of the helper/inducer subset and suppressor cells are known as T8 lymphocytes of the cytotoxic/suppressor subset. Therefore, T4 cells are synonymous with helper cells, while T8 cells are synonymous with suppressor cells.

Figure 3.2 illustrates the inter-relationship between humoral and cell-mediated immunity, and the crucial role played by the helper (T4) cells.

Immune dysfunctions

Survival is impossible without a well-functioning immune system.

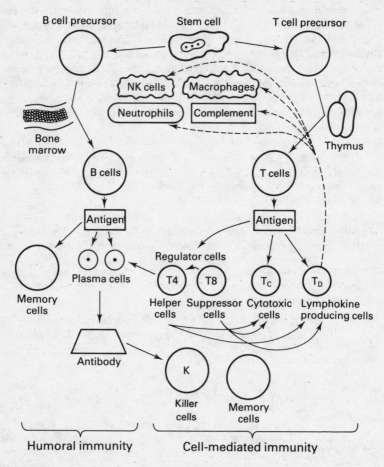

Fig. 3.2   Acquired immunity

However, immune dysfunction is clinically well-recognised. Some children are born with a **primary immune dysfunction**, such as Severe Combined Immunodeficiency [SCID] or DiGeorge Syndrome. In these conditions, fatal flaws in the immune system render the child unable to mount a specific immune response to invading pathogens. The child will die of infectious diseases, which take the opportunity of establishing themselves in a host who is unable to defend himself effectively – hence these infections are referred to as **opportunistic infections**.

Most individuals, however, are born with an effective and fully functional immune system. As life progresses, events and incidents can occur which may depress the immune system, either temporarily or permanently. These are the immunodeficiencies, which are secondary to another cause or condition, i.e. **secondary immunodeficiency**. Secondary immunodeficiencies can be caused by:

Drugs – administration of corticosteroids, immunosuppressants, and most anti-cancer drugs will depress the immune system. During this period, the patient is at increased risk of opportunistic infections, a fact well known to nurses as evidenced by their careful monitoring of patients while on this type of treatment.

Malignant conditions: Hodgkin's disease, leukaemia and other malignancies can cause a severe immunodeficiency.

Protein depletion conditions: Antibodies are made up of protein molecules. Any condition in which there is an inadequate supply of protein in the body, leads to an immunodeficient state. This can be seen in conditions such as the nephrotic syndrome in which there is a renal loss of protein (especially IgG), and in starvation, where inadequate protein renders the individual (often a child) prone to common infections, such as measles, which may then be rapidly fatal.

Radiation: Radiation can depress the bone marrow, affecting its ability to produce the stem cells which eventually become fully mature lymphocytes.

Other conditions: Ageing, debilitation, various infectious diseases, diseases such as sarcoidosis, leprosy, and miliary TB can all cause immunodeficiency, resulting in the individual becoming vulnerable to opportunistic disease.

Immunodeficiency seen in AIDS

AIDS is chiefly, but not exclusively a disorder of cell-mediated immunity. The most striking immunological features seen in AIDS are:

Leukopenia

A reduction in the normal number of white blood cells is accounted for by a severe peripheral **lymphocytopenia**, i.e. a reduction in the numbers of lymphocytes. This reduction in lymphocytes is due to a diminution of helper (T4) cells; suppressor (T8) cells are either unaffected or may increase in number. Regardless, the reduction in helper (T4) cells alters the normal ratio of helper (T4) cells to suppressor (T8) cells (normally 2:1). Not only are helper (T4) cells reduced in number, but they are also functionally defective.

Impaired lymphokine production

There is a defective production of some lymphokines (e.g. interleukin 2 and gamma-interferon).

Defective natural killer cell activity

Although there are normal numbers of circulating NK cells, they are defective. This is related to the decreased production of interferons by lymphokine-producing cells and is probably the chief reason why patients with AIDS are particularly susceptible to Kaposi's sarcoma.

Impaired cytotoxic cell activity

In AIDS, defective cell-mediated cytotoxicity against target cells harbouring viruses is seen. Consequently, patients with AIDS are at increased risk of viral infections.

Defective monocyte function

There is both defective chemotaxis and an impaired ability of monocytes to destroy many pathogens (e.g. *Giardia lamblia, Toxoplasma gondii*).

Polyclonal activation of B-lymphocytes

Although principally a disease of cell-mediated immunity, B-cells are also abnormal, secreting large amounts of non-specific IgG and IgA. As a result, patients with AIDS have elevated levels of gamma-globulin. As the B-cells are functionally defective, the antibody produced is undifferentiated, i.e. faulty and non-specific. Patients with AIDS are not able to develop specific humoral immunity to any new antigens.

Laboratory results in patients with AIDS

There is currently no consistent and reliable laboratory test diagnostic of AIDS. However, the results below are commonly seen:–

(1) Decreased number of lymphocytes
(2) Absolute decrease in T-lymphocytes, especially peripheral blood helper (T4) cells.
(3) A reversal of the usual helper (T4) to suppressor (T8) cell, ratio. Although seen in other illnesses, especially viral conditions, and in some asymptomatic individuals, it is usually attributed to an increase in suppressor (T8) cells; in AIDS it is due to an absolute decrease in helper (T4) cells.
(4) Cutaneous anergy – AIDS patients cannot mount a delayed hypersensitivity response (a function of cell-mediated immunity) on skin testing with various antigens.
(5) Elevated levels of IgG and IgA.
(6) May or may not be positive for antibodies to the AIDS-virus (HIV).

It can be appreciated that perhaps the most devastating immunological defect in patients with AIDS is the absolute reduction in helper (T4) cells. Without the 'help' of these cells, the entire, intricate pattern of the immune system is defective. It is thus easier to understand why patients with AIDS present with opportunistic infections and neoplastic conditions. It is this new understanding of these defects of acquired immunity which is pointing the way for many researchers as they quickly move forward in investigating the treatment of this catastrophic condition[1,2].

References

1. Pinching, A.J. (1984). Review. The Acquired Immune Deficiency Syndrome. *Clinical Experimental Immunology*, 56(1):1–13
2. Fauci, A.S., *et al*. (1985). NIH Conference – The Acquired Immunodeficiency Syndrome: An Update. *Annals of Internal Medicine*. 102:800–13

4

The Means of Transmission

HIV is a blood-borne virus and has been isolated from blood[1], semen[2], saliva[3], tears[4], breast milk[5] and cerebrospinal fluid[6]. It is principally a sexually transmitted disease. However, transmission can occur via a variety of methods involving contact with blood, blood products, and other body fluids, as listed in Table 4.1.

Table 4.1   HIV: means of transmission

1. Sexually, via contact with infected blood and semen, especially (but not exclusively) via homosexual intercourse

2. Following transfusion of blood or blood products from donor blood infected with HIV

3. Intravenous substance abuse – contamination with infected blood through sharing needles and syringes

4. Following organ transplants or artificial insemination by donor semen

5. Transplacental and perinatal transmission

Although the virus has been isolated in saliva, there has been only one documented case of HIV infection being transmitted by this route[7].

Sexual transmission   The chief route of transmission is via sexual activity. Homosexual (and heterosexual) anal intercourse is an efficient means of transmission, due to the presence of both potentially infected semen and small amounts of blood, which are common in penetrative rectal intercourse. In Europe and the United States, homosexual or bisexual men constitute the largest group of individuals who have contracted HIV infection. This is due to the propensity for anal sex and the multiplicity of sexual partners often associated with this group. Heterosexual vaginal intercourse is also a reasonably efficient means of virus transmission, due to both potentially infected semen and vaginal secretions containing infected lymphocytes. In Africa, AIDS is principally a heterosexually spread disease.

Blood and blood products   AIDS has been transmitted following transfusion of whole blood, blood components and the administration of concentrated Factor VIII, manufactured from pooled plasma and used in the treatment of haemophilia. The routine screening of donor blood for the presence of anti-HIV and the self-exclusion of donors from known high risk groups will substantially decrease (but not totally eliminate) infection from this source.

Intravenous substance abuse   Individuals who are addicted to intravenous drugs account for the second largest group of individuals who have contracted HIV infection in the United States. In the UK, cases of AIDS and AIDS-related complex (ARC) are expected to rise significantly in the next few years as it is now known that large numbers of intravenous substance abusers are infected with HIV[8]. Infection is transmitted by sharing blood-contaminated needles and syringes.

Organ transplants and artificial insemination by donor semen   Donor organs (kidneys, corneas, hearts) are a potential risk and individuals in high risk groups for contracting AIDS are advised not to donate organs or to carry donor cards. A further risk with donor organ transplantation is that recipients receive immunosuppressive therapy to prevent rejection and frequently receive blood transfusions during surgery. The routine screening of donors for anti-HIV will diminish this risk substantially. Cases have been reported of recipients of artificial insemination of donor semen acquiring HIV infection[9]. This risk will decrease with screening of donors, the voluntary self-exclusion of donors from known high risk groups, and the exclusive use of cryopreserved donor semen, stored for 3–6 months and not used until the donor has been retested for anti-HIV. The use of fresh semen in artificial insemination programmes will remain a possible risk.

Transplacental and perinatal transmission   AIDS in children was first reported in 1982. By January 13 1986, 231 children in the United States had been diagnosed as suffering from AIDS[10]. Children have contracted HIV infection as a result of receiving blood transfusions or concentrated Factor VIII for haemophilia, or more commonly, as a result of having a parent infected with HIV. Paediatric cases of HIV infection have occurred in the UK and in other European countries. Infection may be contracted in utero, at birth, or in the neonatal period. Most cases result from perinatal transmission of HIV[11, 12]. There has been one documented case of a child, infected by blood transfusions, who transmitted the infection to his mother who frequently became contaminated with blood and body fluids when caring for him[13].

'At risk' groups

In the United States, most cases (73 per cent) of AIDS have occurred in men with homosexual or bisexual orientation (8 per cent of these men have also been intravenous substance abusers) and in heterosexual intravenous substance abusers (17 per cent). Persons with haemophilia and the heterosexual sex partners of persons with AIDS or 'at risk' for AIDS have each accounted for 1 per cent of cases. Recipients of transfused blood or blood components have accounted for 2 per cent of cases and the remaining 6 per cent did not fit into any of these groups[14]. This pattern of defined 'at risk' groups is similiar in the UK and Western Europe, with the exception that a lower proportion of cases have occurred in intravenous substance abusers. As previously mentioned, a sharp increase in this group can be expected within the next two to three years. In Europe, many cases have also originated from individuals who have come from, or have travelled to Africa. Figure 4.1 represents the currently defined known 'at risk' groups, i.e. those presently most vulnerable (at risk) to contracting AIDS.

Sexual transmission of HIV, in both the USA and the UK, is most frequently **male-to-male** and is well documented. **Male-to-female transmission** is also well documented by accounts of HIV infection in women after artificial insemination with donor semen[15] and by haemophiliacs who have passed HIV infection to their wives[16]. Indeed, there is one documented case of a women contracting AIDS as a result of a single episode of vaginal intercourse[17]. **Female-to-male transmission**, occurs[18] as evidenced by the current situation in Africa, where there are equal numbers of men and women infected, and the documentation of clusters of heterosexual cases[19, 20]. Prostitutes, many of whom are intravenous substance abusers, may well become a reservoir of infection and an important 'bridging group' in the future.

Risk factors

The chief risk factor associated with contracting HIV infection is **unprotected, casual sex**. The more sexual partners an individual has, the more likely it is that they will be exposed to various sexually transmitted diseases, including HIV infection. Anal sex (in either homosexuals or heterosexuals) is a significant risk factor associated with this infection, as is contamination with infected blood, such as that encountered by intravenous substance abusers sharing needles and syringes. Table 4.2 summarizes the most important current risk factors known to be associated with this disease.

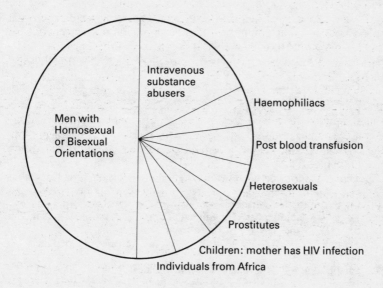

Fig. 4.1 'At risk' groups – USA and Europe

Table 4.2 Important risk factors associated with HIV infection

1. Multiplicity of sexual partners
2. Anal sex
3. Intravenous substance abuse if needles and/or syringes are shared

Although homosexual men were particularly vulnerable to this infection during the early years of the epidemic, AIDS and other manifestations of HIV infection are not exclusive to this group of individuals. All sexually active individuals can be infected, if exposed to the virus under the right circumstances. Nurses have both a unique responsibility and opportunity to assist in the health education efforts currently being implemented by the Health Services aimed at primary prevention. The role of the nurse in patient education as related to HIV infection is discussed in Chapter 7.

References

1. Gallo, R.C., Salahuddin, S.Z., Popovic, M., *et al*. (1984). Frequent detection and isolation of cytopathic retroviruses (HTLV-III) from patients with AIDS and at risk for AIDS. *Science* 224:500-3
2. Zagury, D., Bernard, J., Leibowitch, J., *et al*. (1984). HTLV-III in cells cultured from semen of two patients with AIDS. *Science* 226:449-51
3. Groopman, J.E., Salahuddin, S.Z., Sarngadharan, M.G., *et al*. (1984). HTLV-III in saliva of people with AIDS-related complex and healthy homosexual men at risk for AIDS. *Science* 226:447-9
4. Fujikawa, L.S., Palestine, A.G., Nussenblatt, R.B., *et al*. (1985). Isolation of human T-lymphotropic virus type III from the tears of a patient with the Acquired Immune Deficiency Syndrome. *Lancet*. (September 7) ii(8454):529-30
5. Thirty, L., Sprecher-Goldberger, S., Jonckheer, T., *et al*. (1985). Isolation of AIDS virus from cell-free breast milk of three healthy virus carriers. *Lancet*. (October 19) ii(8460):891-2
6. Levy, J.A., Hollander, H., Shimabukura, J., *et al*. (1985). Isolation of AIDS-associated retroviruses from cerebrospinal fluid and brain of patients with neurological symptoms. *Lancet*. (September 14) ii(8455):586-8
7. Salahuddin, S.Z., Markham, P.D., Redfield, R.R., *et al*. (1984). HTLV-III in symptom-free seronegative persons. *Lancet*. (December 22/29) ii(8417/8):1418-20
8. Robertson, J.R., Bucknall, A.B.V., Welsby, P.D., *et al*. (1986). Epidemic of AIDS related virus (HTLV-III/LAV) infection among intravenous drug abusers. *British Medical Journal* (February 22) 292:527-9
9. Stewart, G.J., Cunningham, A.L., Driscoll, G.L., *et al*. (1985). Transmission of Human T-Cell Lymphotropic Virus Type III (HTLV-III) by artificial insemination by donor. *Lancet*. (September 14) ii(8455):581-4
10. CDC (Centers for Disease Control). (1986). Update: Acquired Immunodeficiency Syndrome - United States. *MMWR* (January 17) 35(2):17
11. Spira, T.J., and Castro, K.G. (1986). The epidemiology of the Acquired Immunodeficiency Syndrome, in *Acquired Immunodeficiency Syndrome* (Progress in Allergy, Vol. 37) ed. by E. Klein. Karger, Basel. p 73

12. CDC (17 January 1986) *op. cit.* p 21
13. CDC (Centers for Disease Control). (1986). Apparent transmission of Human T-Lymphotropic Virus Type III/Lymphadenopathy-Associated Virus from a child to a mother providing health care. *MMWR* 35(5):76–9
14. CDC (17 January 1986) *op. cit.*, p 18
15. Stewart (1985) *loc. cit.*
16. Pitchenik, A.E., Shafron, R.D., Glasser, R.M., *et al.* (1984). The Acquired Immunodeficiency Syndrome in the wife of a hemophiliac. *Annals of Internal Medicine* (January) 100(1):62–5
17. Cabane, J., Thibierge, E., Godeau, P., *et al.* (1984). AIDS in an apparently risk-free woman. *Lancet* (July 14) ii(8394):105
18. Redfield, P.R., Markham, P.D., Salahuddin, S.Z., *et al.* (1985). Heterosexually acquired HTLV-III/LAV disease (AIDS-related complex and AIDS). Epidemiologic evidence for female-to-male transmission. *Journal of the American Medical Association*, (October 18) 254(15):2094–96
19. Clumeck, N., Sonnet, J., Taelman, H., *et al.* (1984). Acquired immunodeficiency syndrome in African patients. *New England Journal of Medicine* (February 23) 310(8):492–7
20. Piot, P., Quinn, T.C., Haelman, H., *et al.* (1984). Acquired immunodeficiency syndrome in a heterosexual population in Zaire. *Lancet* (July 14) ii(8394):65–69L

5

The Presenting Illnesses of Acquired Immunodeficiency Syndrome

A succession of disasters came on him so swiftly and with such unexpected violence that it is hard to say when exactly I recognized that my friend was in deep trouble.

Brideshead Revisited. Evelyn Waugh

Infection with HIV produces three alternatives: perhaps as many as 50 per cent of individuals infected with this retrovirus will remain asymptomatic (at least in the short term, i.e. 5 years) and are known to have been infected only when blood tests for the antibody to HIV (anti-HIV) are positive. However, they remain *infected* and *infectious* (Figure 5.1).

Another 30 per cent will develop **AIDS-related Complex** (ARC); some of these will progress to fully expressed AIDS. Some will stabilize in their relative state of ill-health, and a few may recover.

The remaining 20 per cent of individuals infected with HIV will proceed directly to fully expressed AIDS. In this chapter, we are going to examine the clinical presentation of patients with ARC and AIDS – i.e. the reasons why they are admitted to hospital.

AIDS-related complex

In 1981 many individuals in the same groups becoming known as 'at risk' for fully expressed AIDS were being seen for an equally new syndrome of unexplained, persistent, generalized lymphadenopathy, accompanied by an influenza-like illness with fever, night sweats, weight loss and fatigue. The lymphadenopathy (swollen lymph glands) always involved axillary and cervical lymph nodes and this syndrome became known as either 'Persistent, generalized lymphadenopathy (PGL)' or more commonly, the 'Lymphadenopathy Syndrome (LAS)'. Many variations of this syndrome were seen and some, but not all, of these men additionally presented with an enlarged spleen (splenomegaly), a reduction in white blood cells (leukopenia), and abnormalities of the immune system (e.g. decrease in total numbers of helper (T4)

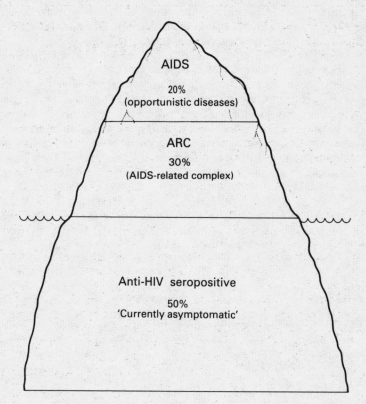

Fig. 5.1 The clinical spectrum of HIV infection

cells, hence a decrease in the (T4) helper: (T8) suppressor cell ratio, cutaneous anergy to many recall skin test antigens, and elevated levels of gamma globulin). In addition, most had serological evidence of past exposure to various viruses, e.g. **cytomegalovirus** (CMV), **Epstein-Barr virus, herpes simplex** and **hepatitis B** virus. Thrombocytopenia and oral candidiasis (thrush) were seen in some of these men and lymph node biopsy usually demonstrated a follicular hyperplasia commonly seen in lymph glands following acute viral infections.

Some men also presented with white, elevated lesions on the side of the tongue known as hairy leukoplakia (HL). All the variations in ill-health seen between asymptomatic sero-positive individuals and fully expressed AIDS have become known as **AIDS-related Complex (ARC)**.

It is difficult to predict which of these individuals with ARC will progress to fully expressed AIDS but LAS, with constitutional symptoms, splenomegaly, leukopenia, and lymph nodes displaying follicular hyperplasia, are generally predictive of progression to AIDS, as is the presence of hairy leukoplakia.

Many patients with the signs and symptoms of ARC will be admitted to hospital for investigations, which may include a lymph node biopsy under a general anaesthetic. They are usually relatively well, fully ambulatory, requiring the minimum of nursing care. Patients with ARC, unlike those with AIDS, do not have overt opportunistic infections. They may, however, have a variety of minor skin infections and some have seborrheic dermatitis. Latent viral conditions may be reactivated in patients with ARC and recurrent genital herpes, genital warts and herpes zoster may be seen. A few patients with ARC may develop oral candidiasis. Idiopathic diarrhoea is also seen in some patients. ARC is best seen as a milder response to infection with HIV on an ascending ladder leading to a profound, progressive and persistent immunodeficiency resulting in fully expressed AIDS with opportunistic infections and/or neoplastic conditions.

AIDS

Patients are admitted to hospital for a variety of opportunistic infections associated with this syndrome. They are called 'opportunistic' as they are infections caused by pathogens which the body, in health, contains quite easily. However, in AIDS, these pathogens have taken the 'opportunity' of a depressed immune system to establish clinical illness. Although it is possible for a patient to be admitted with just one infectious disease, patients with AIDS more commonly present with a host of infections. We will look at each individually, remembering then that they frequently occur together in various combinations (Table 5.1).

Table 5.1   Opportunistic pathogens seen in HIV infection

Protozoal Infections
  Pneumocystis carinii
  Toxoplasma gondii
  Cryptosporidium species
  Giardia lamblia
  Entamoeba histolytica
  Isospora species

Bacterial Infections
    Mycobacterium tuberculosis
    Mycobacterium avium-intracellulare
    Mycobacterium kanasii/xenopi
    Salmonella typhimurium
    Shigella flexneri
    Legionella species
    Listeria monocytogenes
    Norcardia species

Fungal Infections
    Candida albicans
    Cryptococcus neoformans
    Aspergillus species
    Coccidioides immitis
    Tinea species

Viral Infections
    Cytomegalovirus
    Herpes simplex
    Herpes zoster
    Epstein-Barr virus
    Papova viruses (JC/SV-40)

Pneumocystis carinii pneumonia (PCP)

PCP (also referred to as 'pneumocystosis') is not only the main present-ing disease seen in AIDS, it is by far the most frequent cause of death in persons with AIDS. The organism, first described in 1909, is a multi-flagellate protozoan and was first recognised as a human pathogen during World War II when it caused a fatal pneumonia in severely mal-nourished refugee children. *P. carinii* is part of the normal flora of most adults, rarely causing disease unless the immune system becomes com-promised. In the United States, the first case of pneumonia in an adult caused by *P. carinii* was observed in 1954. Until the present epidemic of AIDS, PCP was only seen in patients whose immune system had been depressed by either a known primary or secondary cause, e.g. congeni-tal immunodeficiency disorders, or patients receiving chemotherapy for cancer, or immunosuppressant drugs following transplant surgery. It is a relatively important point for the nurse to note that PCP only occurs in immunocompromised individuals; hence hospital personnel and other patients, who are not immunocompromised, are not at risk of acquiring this infection.

Patients usually develop symptoms insidiously, often giving a three to four week history of cough, dyspnoea, chest pain, fever and chills. Tachypnoea (rapid respirations) and cyanosis are usually present when the patient is seen in hospital.

Some patients have a more fulminate course with a much shorter history. The patient may be in acute respiratory failure and in extreme distress.

The diagnosis of PCP is difficult. All the usual causes of pneumonia will need to be excluded and sputum will be obtained for routine culture and sensitivity (sputum specimens, useful for establishing the aetiology of many types of pneumonia, are not helpful in diagnosing PCP). Chest X-rays usually show alveolar and interstitial infiltrates in both the right and left lung field (bilateral). These changes however, may be so mild as to be interpreted as normal in many patients. Abnormalities of arterial blood gases (associated with hypoxaemia) are common. The diagnosis of PCP is generally made as a result of bronchoalveolar lavage of sub-segmental bronchi, or transbronchial biopsy, both distressing procedures in patients with an already established respiratory impairment. Bronchoscopy is often carried out in the patient's room using a 'dedicated' instrument reserved for patients with this disease. Biopsy can also help diagnose co-existing pulmonary infection with mycobacterium, CMV or *Cryptococcus neoformans*.

Once PCP has been diagnosed, treatment is initiated with either pentamidine isethionate or trimethoprim-sulfamethoxazole ('Bactrim,' 'Septrin').

Pentamidine isethionate – this drug is usually administered intramuscularly in a dose of 4 mg/kg., once daily for at least 21 days.

Side effects – almost half of all patients receiving pentamidine experience side effects, ranging from nephrotoxicity (with elevated creatinine levels), hypoglycaemia (and sometimes, hyperglycaemia), sterile abscesses at the injection site, disorders of blood clotting (e.g. thrombocytopenia), skin rashes and pruritus (severe itching), tachycardia and hypotension. The abscesses at the injection site may become secondarily infected, providing yet another focus of infection for this immunocompromised patient and can be so painful that the patient may refuse further injections. Intramuscular injections into a wasted, catabolic patient present nursing care problems and although using alternative sites is helpful, the formation of abscesses, or the bleeding disorders sometimes caused by this drug, may preclude it being used intramuscularly.

For these reasons, intravenous administration of pentamidine is becoming more common. Pentamidine, diluted in at least 100 ml of 5 per cent dextrose/water, is given slowly (over 1–2 hours), once daily, under close supervision, as this route of administration has been associated with intractable hypotension.

Nursing implications of pentamidine therapy – urine specimens should be tested and blood glucose levels measured daily. Arterial blood pressure should be taken and recorded four hourly, unless unstable, when it should be taken more frequently. During intravenous administrations of pentamidine, the blood pressure should be taken every 15 minutes.

Trimethoprim-sulfamethoxazole – also known as 'co-trimoxazole', is given in high doses (e.g. 20 mg. trimethoprim/100 mg sulfamethoxazole/kg) either orally or intravenously, in divided doses, every eight hours, again for at least 21 days. Although generally this drug is associated with fewer side effects than pentamidine, a high percentage of patients with AIDS (up to 65 per cent) develop a drug fever, rash and significant leukopenia when treated with this compound. Side effects may be controlled by the administration of antihistamines, and/or by giving trimethoprim separately and reducing the dose of sulfonamide. Intravenous infusions should be run in slowly (over one and a half hours) and care should be taken not to mistake **intramuscular** preparations for intravenous use. When given orally, nausea, vomiting and diarrhoea are not uncommon. It is usual for the medical staff to prescribe folinic acid (calcium folinate) 15 mg two to three times weekly in an attempt to prevent the bone marrow depression due to high dose trimethoprim-sulfamethoxazole therapy; this may be given orally or intravenously.

Although, in theory, long term prophylaxis with trimethoprim-sulfamethoxazole would be useful, it rarely can be used as such, due to the considerable number of patients who experience intolerable side effects from it.

Other drugs used include – DFMO (alpha difluoromethylorinthine), sulfadoxine and pyrimethamine ('Fansidar') and Dapsone. These drugs are anti-parasitic and side effects associated with them include haematological abnormalities, nephrotoxicity and nausea and vomiting.

Improvement, if it is to be seen, usually occurs within five to ten days. Although perhaps as many as 70 per cent of patients with AIDS who present with PCP can be successfully treated with the above drugs, they will eventually return to hospital with another episode, more difficult to treat. The long-term survival rate in patients, who have AIDS and present with PCP, is poor; the median cumulative survival is approximately 35 weeks. The quality of life is also poor with many patients (up to 40 per cent) spending more than half the time from date of diagnosis until death, in hospital.

Other causes of pneumonia in AIDS

The somewhat aggressive investigations required to diagnose PCP are needed, not only because the drugs used to treat this pneumonia are relatively toxic, hence the physician wants to be sure he actually is treating *P. carinii*, but also because several other opportunistic pathogens, some of which are treatable, are also known to cause pneumonia in patients with AIDS. These include mycobacteria (i.e. pulmonary tuberculosis and pneumonia caused by *Mycobacterium avium intracellulare*), bacteria (e.g. *Streptococcus pneumoniae* and *Haemophilus influenzae*), viruses (e.g. *CMV* and *herpes simplex*), fungi (*aspergillus* and *cryptococcus*) and protozoa (e.g. *Toxoplasma gondii*), plus Kaposi's sarcoma, which involves the lungs in some patients.

Mycobacterial infections are treated with anti-tuberculosis drugs such as rifampicin, ethambutol, isoniazid, and newer agents such as ansamycin and clofazimine, although the response to treatment is poor. Bacterial infections are treated with the appropriate antibiotics as indicated by culture and sensitivity, and other therapies are available for some of the varied agents, which can cause pneumonia in the patient with AIDS. Bronchoalveolar lavage allows the physician to culture many of these opportunists and transbronchial biopsy (or open lung biopsy) can demonstrate pulmonary involvement of Kaposi's sarcoma.

Toxoplasmosis

Toxoplasmosis is caused by a small, intracellular protozoan parasite, *Toxoplasma gondii*. This parasite is found in most animals (especially pet cats) and man is often asymptomatically infected. It is only when the immune system fails to keep this parasite in check that it is able to cause clinical illness. In patients with AIDS, *T. gondii* can cause a variety of clinical disorders, but the most common illness seen related to infection with this agent is toxoplasma encephalitis.

Patients with toxoplasma encephalitis frequently present with neurological signs such as confusion, headache, vertigo and seizures. The patient often has an elevated temperature and is lethargic. The various signs and symptoms may resemble those seen in space-occupying lesions of the brain or those following stroke. The patient is seriously ill and can deteriorate with alarming speed.

Although encephalitis is by far the most frequent manifestation of toxoplasmosis in patients with AIDS, pneumonia and/or myocarditis can also occur.

In toxoplasma encephalitis, X-rays, CT scans, lumbar punctures and serological blood tests are usually abnormal, but changes seen are nonspecific and the diagnosis is made by brain biopsy.

Once diagnosed, treatment is initiated with pyrimethamine and sulfadiazine. The usual doses used are: pyrimethamine – loading dose of 75 mg orally and then 25 mg orally, each day. Sulfadiazine – 1 gram orally or intravenously, four times daily. Folinic acid (calcium folinate) 15 mg, three times weekly, is often concurrently prescribed to prevent the serious consequences of depressed folate metabolism associated with pyrimethamine, e.g. leukopenia, thrombocytopenia and anaemia.

Other drugs used to treat toxoplasma encephalitis include clindamycin and spiramycin. Corticosteroids and anticonvulsants may also be prescribed.

As it is impossible to eradicate *T. gondii* completely, treatment with these powerful drugs may have to continue for the remaining length of the patient's life.

Cryptosporidiosis

The protozoan, *Cryptosporidia*, has been recognised only in the last ten years as a potential human pathogen, causing a self-limited diarrhoea in animal workers (e.g. veterinarians and slaughterhouse workers). It is spread by a faecal-oral route and, in the immuno-deficient individual, attacks the intestines (principally the small intestines), causing abdominal cramps, fever, nausea and vomiting and a profuse diarrhoea. In AIDS, this can be a catastrophic complication – diarrhoea can range from 3–4 bowel movements a day, to patients passing large amounts (10–12 litres/day) of watery diarrhoea, becoming hypotensive and showing signs and symptoms of electrolyte imbalance. This wasting, weakening disease attacks not only the small bowel, but also the patient's self-esteem, causing psychological havoc.

The diagnosis is made by using special techniques of staining smears of stool specimens or by biopsy of the gastrointestinal mucosa.

At the present time there is no specific therapy which is curative for this infection. Treatment with a macrolide antibiotic known as spiramycin ('Rovamycin' – May and Baker, 250 mg tablets) has been useful in some cases. It is given as one gram, three times daily for 1 to 16 weeks.

Supportive treatment includes antidiarrhoeals, such as loperamide hydrochloride ('Imodium') and diphenoxylate hydrochloride with atropine sulphate ('Lomotil'), rehydration, electrolyte replacement, and nutritional support.

Diarrhoea is seen in most patients with AIDS and only in some is *Cryptosporidia* the cause. Other causes include **amoebiasis** (caused by the protozoan – *Entamoeba histolytica*) and **giardiasis** (caused by another protozoan, *Giardia lamblia*). These are not uncommon enteric infections in homosexuals and the diarrhoea seen is generally less than that seen in cryptosporidiosis. Amoebiasis is treated with oral metronidazole ('Flagyl') and diiodohydroxyquin, and giardiasis is treated with atabrine or metronidazole.

Salmonellosis (caused by salmonellas), may be seen in AIDS as yet another opportunistic cause of diarrhoea. Most strains of salmonella species cause a self-limiting diarrhoea, requiring only supportive treatment; some strains may cause severe disease (e.g. typhoid fever) and require specific treatment with either ampicillin or chloramphenicol. Other opportunists associated with diarrhoea in patients with AIDS include *Shigella*, *Isospora belli*, *Campylobacter*, *Microsporidia* and *Mycobacterium avium-intracellulare*. Kaposi's sarcoma may be an additional cause. Diarrhoea is perhaps one of the most distressing complications of AIDS, and often one of the most difficult to treat.

Mycobacterial infections

There are two mycobacterial diseases associated with AIDS. The first one is *Mycobacterium avium-intracellulare* – a common potential pathogen that in the past rarely caused disease in man, even when immunocompromised. However, it is frequently seen as disseminated disease in patients with AIDS and presents as a disease similar to pulmonary tuberculosis. The disease then quickly disseminates to most organs in the body (spleen, bone marrow, lymph nodes, gastrointestinal tract, skin, and the brain), producing varied signs and symptoms, depending on which part of the body it was causing the most destruction. Patients generally have fever and chills, weight loss and fatigue.

Another mycobacterium sometimes associated with a lung condition similar to tuberculosis is *Mycobacterium kansasii*, which may also cause disseminated disease, cutaneous abscesses, bone and joint involvement, lymphadenitis and meningitis. Person-to-person transmission does not occur with either *M. avium-intracellulare* or *M. kansasii*.

Mycobacterium tuberculosis causes pulmonary tuberculosis. Once the patient is immunocompromised, latent infections commonly flare up to produce active disease and as a result, pulmonary tuberculosis is seen in some patients with AIDS.

The diagnosis of mycobacterial infection involves biopsies of infected organs, chest X-rays, and blood and sputum cultures.

Although pulmonary tuberculosis usually can be controlled with routine anti-tuberculosis therapy, *Mycobacterium avium-intracellulare* and *M. kansasii* are highly resistant to treatment. Various combinations of drugs may be tried, including clofazimine and ansamycin.

Cryptococcal infection

Infection caused by the fungus *Cryptococcosis neoformans* (also known as *Filobasidiella neoformans*), a ubiquitous organism in nature, mainly causes meningitis in immunocompromised individuals. It can affect other areas in the body (e.g. lungs, bone, and the genito-urinary system) and prior to the current epidemic of AIDS was seen mainly in individuals with Hodgkin's disease.

Patients with AIDS may present with a slowly developing meningitis, complaining of headache, mild pyrexia and sometimes blurred vision. Other neurological signs and symptoms associated with meningitis (e.g. positive Kernig's sign, confusion, changes in level of consciousness, etc.) may develop, and the patient may become nauseated and start vomiting.

Cryptococcal meningitis is diagnosed by finding the fungus in cerebrospinal fluid, sputum, urine and blood cultures.

Drugs used for treating this severe infection include **amphotericin B** and **5-flucytosine**. Flucytosine may further depress the white cell count and also cause thrombocytopenia. Treatment is usually given for 10–12 weeks, but relapse is common once treatment finishes.

Viral infections – Herpesviruses

Patients with AIDS are particularly prone to infection with, or re-activation of, various herpesviruses, the most significant being cytomegaloviruses (CMV), herpes simplex viruses, varicella-zoster virus, and Epstein-Barr virus.

Cytomegalovirus infection

As children and young adults, most of us will have been exposed to **cytomegaloviruses** ('CMV'), a common, air-borne spread group of viruses ('salivary gland viruses'). CMV infection may also occur congenitally, postnatally, and can be acquired following blood transfusion ('Post-Perfusion Syndrome'). Infection with CMV produces variable results. Most infants infected show no clinical disease, but congenitally acquired CMV infection may cause abortion, stillbirth, postnatal death, or severe central nervous system damage. In children and adults who acquire this infection, most are asymptomatic, and a few may develop a mononucleosis or hepatitis. CMV are ubiquitous and 60 to 90 per cent of adults will have been exposed to this virus group and will have developed antibodies. When infected with CMV, individuals will excrete this virus in urine, saliva, cervical secretions, semen, faeces and breast milk for several months. Eventually, the process of cell-mediated immunity contains the infection, the individual developing a **latent infection**, and in most cases, never being aware that he or she had been infected in the first place. Like other latent infections normally contained by the immune system, in AIDS, CMV infection becomes re-activated as cell-mediated immunity is destroyed by the AIDS virus.

Most AIDS patients will have re-activated CMV infection and usually are viremic (i.e. have virus in their blood). In the constellation of opportunistic infections seen in patients with AIDS, it is often difficult to establish just what the clinical consequences of re-activated CMV infection are. However, as it may cause ulcerations of the gastro-intestinal tract, it may be implicated as yet another cause of diarrhoea seen in these patients. CMV can cause a terminal **pneumonitis** and also causes a **retinochoroiditis** which may lead to blindness.

Effective treatment for CMV infection has been unsatisfactory. New drugs currently being tried such as **DHPG** (Syntex Corporation), **B759U** (Burroughs-Wellcome Company) and **Phosphonoformate** (**'Foscarnet'** – Astra Pharmaceuticals) are reported to show good results.

Herpes simplex virus infection

Many adults (including a large proportion of homosexual men) have been exposed to **herpes simplex** and consequently harbour these latent viruses. In AIDS they are frequently re-activated and may cause severe **perineal or facial lesions**. They will usually respond to treatment with the antiviral drug, **acyclovir**.

Other viral infections

Many other latent viruses can be re-activated in AIDS and they include:

Varicella-zoster virus – causes herpes zoster (shingles) and is generally seen in patients with AIDS-related complex. Its occurrence may be prognostic of progression to fully expressed AIDS. These lesions respond to intravenous acyclovir, although oral acyclovir may have to be continued indefinitely to prevent relapse. This virus may also cause chickenpox (varicella) in non-immune individuals.

Epstein-Barr virus – may cause fever, lassitude and lymphadenopathy in patients with AIDS. There is no specific treatment available for illness associated with this virus.

Candidal species infection

Infection with **candidal species fungi** in healthy adults is now often associated as being a harbinger of AIDS. Most patients with AIDS have oral candidiasis ('thrush'), often affecting the oesophagus and rectum. Disseminated candidiasis can occur, but it is usually associated with indwelling catheters or prolonged treatment with antibiotics. Although sometimes responsive to treatment with nystatin or clotrimazole, candidiasis is frequently resistant to these agents. In such cases, ketoconazole or amphotericin B are usually effective. Candida oesophagitis is serious and may cause perforation and haemorrhage. Treatment with the above agents has to be continued for the remainder of the patient's life as, if discontinued, relapse is invariable.

Other opportunistic pathogens in AIDS

Although the opportunistic conditions we have discussed are the ones most frequently seen as a manifestation of immunodeficiency in patients with AIDS, and serve to define this disease, they are by no means the only potential pathogens which take the opportunity to establish clinical disease in the absence of immune competence. Other opportunists which may be encountered include:

Isospora belli – may cause severe diarrhoea

Histoplasma capsulatum – causes *histoplasmosis*, a progressive, disseminating fungal disease involving lungs, spleen, liver and the gastrointestinal tract

Coccidioides immitis – causes *coccidiodomycosis*, another disseminated fungal disease involving many organs in the body including the brain, and may be involved in causing meningitis

Nocardia asteroides – causes *nocardiosis*, a disseminating disease associated with metastatic brain abscesses, skin or subcutaneous abscesses and pulmonary lesions

Listeria monocytogenes – causes *listeriosis*, meningitis being its most frequent clinical presentation

Papova viruses – JC virus and SV-40 virus have been implicated in causing a severe, progressive, demyelinating disease in patients with AIDS, known as *progressive multifocal leukoencephalopathy (PML)*. This is a rare but serious infection of the central nervous system for which there is no effective therapy at present.

All patients with AIDS will develop opportunistic infection at some time during the course of their illness. Even though some, such as *P. carinii* pneumonia, are treatable, eventually they become more difficult, if not impossible, to treat and eventually, after incapacitating illness, cause death in patients with AIDS.

The other remaining major opportunistic disease seen in AIDS is Kaposi's sarcoma.

Kaposi's sarcoma

Prior to the current epidemic of AIDS, Kaposi's sarcoma (KS) was a relatively unusual vascular tumour, first described by a Hungarian dermatologist, Moriz Kaposi, in 1872. In the United States and in Western Europe, Kaposi's sarcoma was mainly seen in elderly men, especially those of Italian or Eastern European Jewish ancestry, and was relatively benign in its clinical course. Patients presented with discoloured patches, plaques, or nodular skin lesions, brown, red or blue in colour, usually confined to lower extremities (especially the ankles and soles of the feet). These lesions are the result of a multicentric tumour arising from local hyperplasia of a cell of the vascular endothelium. Often, as the patients were in the age group 60–79 years, no specific treatment was indicated. This type of indolent, non-aggressive, non-invasive Kaposi's sarcoma has become known as **classic** Kaposi's sarcoma.

Another form of Kaposi's sarcoma was known to exist in Equatorial Africa, where it was more common. Four different types of Kaposi's sarcoma have been described in Africa, one of which is similar to classic Kaposi's sarcoma, the remaining three being more aggressive, rapidly progressive neoplastic conditions, affecting young African men, often fatal within a year. This African form of Kaposi's sarcoma is sometimes referred to as **endemic** Kaposi's sarcoma.

Prior to 1981, a type of Kaposi's sarcoma similar to the African endemic form was observed in renal patients following kidney transplant and iatrogenic immunosuppression. This too was aggressive, but responded well to discontinuation of immunosuppression therapy and restoration of the patient to immune competence.

With the advent of AIDS in 1981, an aggressive form of Kaposi's sarcoma, similar to African endemic Kaposi's sarcoma, was seen in young, previously healthy male homosexuals. This AIDS-associated Kaposi's sarcoma has become known as **epidemic** Kaposi's sarcoma and patients usually present with asymptomatic, pigmented skin lesions which may be on any part of the body. Lesions can usually be identified in the mouth, especially on the hard palate, and many will also have lymph node enlargement. The initial lesions are multifocal at time of diagnosis, often involving visceral organs (e.g. lungs, liver, spleen, gastrointestinal tract), and rapidly disseminate, usually in an orderly fashion.

The average life expectancy of patients with AIDS who have Kaposi's sarcoma is about 16 months, only a quarter of all patients surviving for two years or more.

Treatment does not improve survival, or the rate of the appearance of new lesions. However, it is useful for palliation and various treatment modalities can be effectively used.

Local irradiation therapy – skin and oral lesions are often radiosensitive and doses under 20 Gy are used.

Chemotherapy – various anti-cancer drugs have been tried and currently the following have been found to be the most useful: *Vinblastine* (given intravenously, once weekly in doses of 4–10 mg). This regime is associated with minimal toxicity and approximately 40 per cent of patients treated may show objective improvement. *VP-16 (epidophyllotoxin)* (given intravenously for 3 days every 3–4 weeks in doses of 150 mg per square metre of body surface). Most patients will experience side effects, especially leukopenia and alopecia; however up to 75 per cent may show objective improvement.

One of the dangers of anti-cancer chemotherapy is the risk of further depressing the immune system and rendering the patient more prone to opportunistic infection. The use of VP-16 is not only associated with the highest objective response rate, but is also associated with the lowest rate of occurrence of opportunistic infection (seen in only 12 per cent of patients treated, as opposed to 25 per cent of patients treated with vinblastine).

Immune modulators – it seemed clear from the beginning of the epidemic that curative treatment for epidemic Kaposi's sarcoma would be available only if immune competence was restored, and various immune modulators have been used in combination with anti-cancer chemotherapy. **Alpha interferons** have been widely used to stimulate the immune system in patients with AIDS and may be useful in treating epidemic Kaposi's sarcoma. However this has not been shown to restore immune competence. Intravenous administration has been shown to be associated with the fewest side effects, which commonly include fever, malaise, headache, and transient, mild confusion. **Gamma interferon** and **interleukin 2** are also being investigated. A serious reservation regarding the use of lymphokines such as the above, is that they may cause proliferation of AIDS-virus infected lymphocytes.

Other tumours in AIDS

Although Kaposi's sarcoma is by far the most common malignancy seen in AIDS, **undifferentiated lymphomas**, affecting various sites including the central nervous system, bone marrow and gastrointestinal tract, may be seen. An increased incidence of other tumours may also be encountered. It may be that the various viruses present in patients with AIDS, or in the major 'at risk' group for AIDS, are potentially oncogenic and once the immune system has broken down, may become involved in the pathogenesis of the various tumours seen.

Summary

Fully expressed AIDS is an acquired immunodeficiency state in which individuals develop one or more opportunistic infections, usually due to latent, potential pathogens which are ubiquitous in nature and which, were it not for the underlying immune deficiency, would not be dangerous. The most common opportunistic infection seen is pneumonia, caused by the protozoan, *P. carinii*. The depressed immune state also involves a breakdown in the normal tumour surveillance carried out by activated natural killer cells and opportunistic cancers are also seen, chiefly Kaposi's sarcoma.

Treatment for either opportunistic infectious diseases or cancers is not curative as the principal defect is in the immune system and, until a way can be found to restore the competence of this system, AIDS will continue to be a fatal disease.

Further reading

McI Johnson, N. (1985). Pneumonia in the acquired immune deficiency syndrome. *British Medical Journal* (May). 290:4:1299–1301

Masur, H. *et al.* (1985). Infectious complications of AIDS, in *AIDS, etiology, diagnosis, treatment and prevention*, ed. by Devita, V., Hellman, S., Rosenberg, S. J.B. Lippincott Co. pp 161–84

Volberding, P. (1984). Therapy of Kaposi's sarcoma in AIDS. *Seminars in Oncology* (March) 11(1):60–67

Ziegler, J.L. and Abrams, D.I. (1985). The AIDS-Related Complex, in *AIDS, etiology, diagnosis, treatment and prevention. op. cit.* pp 223–33

6

The Rationale for Strategic Nursing Care

Patients admitted for investigation or treatment of HIV infection and associated opportunistic disease may be in a rapidly changing clinical situation. Therefore nursing care must be assessed, planned and evaluated on a daily basis. This requires a comprehensive understanding by the nurse of the rationale which underpins strategic nursing care.

Strategic nursing care is that care which is developed and implemented by Registered Nurses, designed to meet the immediate needs of patients, solve identified actual problems and prevent recognised potential problems from being realized. Because of their training and experience, their comprehensive understanding of the nursing issues involved, their teaching and management skills, Registered Nurses are able to assess and plan the individualized nursing care most appropriate for each patient, leading and supervising the nursing team implementing this care. Care delivered must be evaluated frequently (often on a shift-by-shift basis) and modified according to the patient's response to nursing intervention. The Registered Nurse is ideally placed to act as the patient's advocate and to liaise effectively between the patient and other members of the health care team.

It is axiomatic that in assessing and planning strategic nursing care for patients with an infectious disease, an extensive understanding of appropriate infection control (IC) procedures is required.

Virus fragility

There is nothing indestructible about HIV. It can easily be destroyed by a variety of physical and chemical means.

Heat: HIV, like other retroviruses, is readily inactivated by heat. In the presence of normal human serum, HIV is completely inactivated when incubated at a temperature of 56 degrees Celsius (Centigrade) for 30 minutes[1,2]. This is, of course, well below boiling point and any techniques which achieve this temperature (or a higher temperature), are able to inactivate the virus. This includes boiling and autoclaving instruments. Dishwashers and washing machines on a hot cycle will also destroy the virus. In hospital, all non-disposable instruments are sterilized by saturated steam in an autoclave at 2.2 bar, 134 degrees Celsius, maintained for a minimum of 3 minutes[2]. Disposable used instruments, which cannot be incinerated or otherwise sterilized, are autoclaved before being discarded[2]. Incineration of infected dressings and rubbish is usually arranged.

Chemical disinfectants: Standard solutions of almost all common disinfectants destroy the virus[3]. The most effective are:

(1) *sodium hypochlorite* (bleach): one of the most effective (and economical) disinfectants active against HIV is a *freshly* prepared solution of sodium hypochlorite. Strong concentrations contain 10 000 parts per million (ppm) of available chlorine (household bleach, diluted 1 part bleach to 10 parts water)[2, 4, 5].

(2) *glutaraldehyde*: freshly prepared 2% glutaraldehyde is equally effective against HIV. This agent is the active ingredient in a variety of disinfectants, e.g. Asep, Cidex and Totacide[2, 4, 5, 6, 7].

(3) *other disinfectants*: a 25% ethanol solution is also effective in disinfecting medical instruments. Any approved hospital disinfectant, which is 'mycobactericidal' (i.e. tuberculocidal), is equally effective. Standard solutions of hydrogen peroxide, some phenolics, and saponified cresol solutions are also effective agents. Handwashing, using halogenated soaps, appears to eradicate the organism[14]. The virus is also inactivated by exposure to solutions which have a high or low pH[2, 3].

Agents not effective: include 0.1% formalin (which is too slow-acting), gamma irradiation and doses of ultraviolet radiation usually employed under laminar hoods, in operating theatres, or in laboratories[1, 4].

HIV and infection control (IC) procedures

There are two alternative systems of IC precautions: (1) **Category-specific**, and (2) **Disease-specific**. **Category-specific** includes several categories of isolation (Category A, Category B, etc.), depending on the infectiveness, ease and common routes of transmission of **groups** of diseases. The measures taken range from strict isolation to standard IC precautions. The appropriate precautions ('enteric precautions,' 'respiratory precautions,' etc.) are specified on different colour-coded cards, designed for each category. Although this system works well, it has not been found adequate for patients with HIV infections, who present with combinations of different opportunistic diseases.

Disease-specific IC precautions are more flexible. A single card is completed by the nurse, who chooses from a list of the appropriate precautions to be taken, which is relevant for *each* disease.

Figure 6.1 shows an example of a card which is completed for each patient, and displayed prominently.

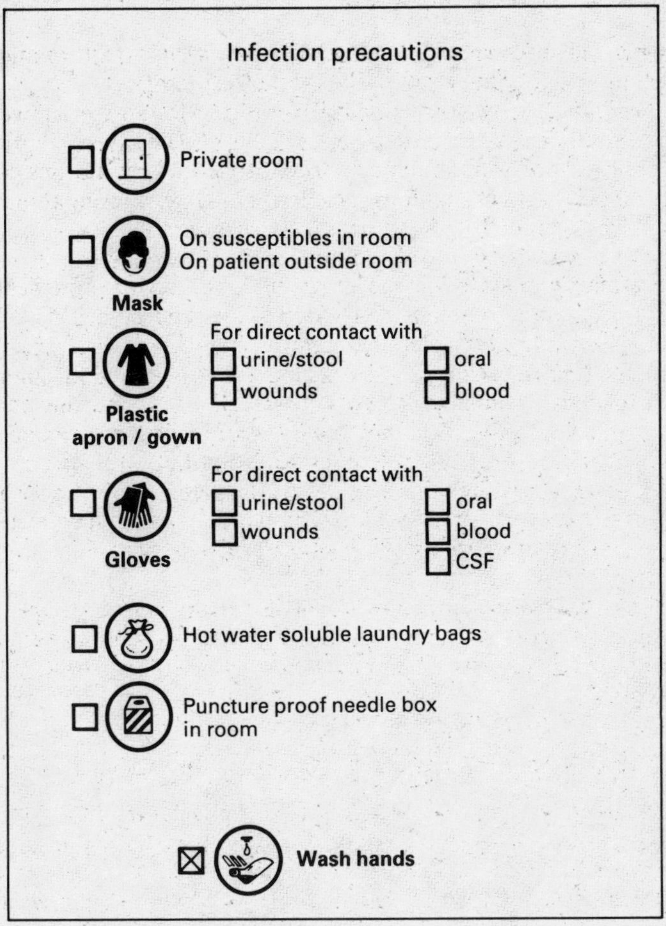

Fig. 6.1 Infection Control precautions card

Disease-specific IC precautions allow individualized nursing care to be modified frequently, according to the changing clinical status of the patient. Table 6.1 summarizes the recommendations for the opportunistic diseases commonly encountered in patients with HIV-related infections.

Table 6.1   Disease specific IC precautions for infections commonly associated with patients who have AIDS

Infection	Single room	Plastic apron	Gloves	Masks	Infective material
AIDS	Only when indicated as per Table 6.3	Yes	Yes	No	Blood and body fluids
ARC	No	Yes	Yes	No	Blood and body fluids
HIV seropositive (asymptomatic)	No	Yes	Yes	No	Blood and body fluids
Amebiasis (dysentery)	Yes, if patient hygiene poor	Yes if soiling likely	Yes if soiling likely	No	Faeces
Candidiasis	No	No	Yes for mouth care	No	Oral secretions
Varicella (chicken pox)	Yes	Yes	Yes	Yes	Respiratory secretions & lesion secretions

NB Nurses who have not had varicella should not nurse patients who have this infection

Infection	Single room	Plastic apron	Gloves	Masks	Infective material
Cryptococcosis	No	No	No	No	
Cryptosporidiosis	Yes for convenience	Yes	Yes	No	Faeces
Cytomegalovirus	No	No	No	No only if coughing excessively	Urine and respiratory secretions may be
Diarrhoea	Yes, if patient	Yes	Yes	No	Faeces

Table 6.1 *Cont'd*

Infection	Single room	Plastic apron	Gloves	Masks	Infective material
	hygiene poor, or for convenience				
EBV Infection	No	No	No	No	Respiratory secretions may be
Giardiasis	Yes for convenience	Yes	Yes	No	Faeces
Salmonella infections	Yes for convenience	Yes	Yes	No	Faeces
Viral hepatitis	Yes, if patient hygiene poor, or if positive for HB 'e' antigen	Yes	Yes	No	Hepatitis A: faeces Hepatitis B: blood and body fluids Hepatitis non-A, non-B: blood and body fluids
Herpes simplex virus infection (mucocutaneous, disseminated or severe skin, oral, or genital) primary or recurrent	Yes	Yes	Yes	No	lesion secretions from infected sites
Herpes Zoster	Yes	Yes	Yes	Yes	lesion secretion and possibly respiratory secretions

NB Nurses who have not had varicella should not care for patients with this infection

continued

Table 6.1 *Cont'd*

Infection	Single room	Plastic apron	Gloves	Masks	Infective material
Mycobacterial infections:					
Atypical (*M.avium-intracellulare*) disseminated or pulmonary	No	No	No	No	
Pulmonary tuberculosis	Yes	Yes	No	Yes	Airborne droplet nuclei
Nocardiosis	No	No	No	No	Draining lesions may be
Legionnaires' disease	No	No	No	No	
Pneumocystis carinii pneumonia	Yes	No	No	Only if coughing excessively	Respiratory secretions
Toxoplasmosis	No	No	No	No	
Coccidiodomycosis	No	No	No	No	
Histoplasmosis	No	No	No	No	
Listeriosis	No	No	No	No	

HIV and general IC precautions

AIDS and AIDS-related conditions are *not* highly infectious in a nursing care setting. The following discussion of general IC precautions related to this condition is in agreement with the guidelines published both in the United Kingdom and the United States of America[8, 9, 10, 11]. These precautions are designed to prevent acquisition of HIV infection by health care workers and to prevent the spread of HTLV-III infection and related opportunistic diseases to other patients. The remote risk of infection to nursing personnel is reduced to zero if these guidelines are followed. In addition they encapsulate competent nursing practice already in existence, which has been designed to care safely for patients with infectious diseases. All nurses have a responsibility to examine and improve their practice constantly and to keep up-to-date with current developments, which may affect their patients. The following general guidelines may be adapted for all patients with AIDS, ARC and asymptomatic HIV infection.

All patients with AIDS, ARC and those who are known to be anti-HIV positive, should be placed on **'Blood/Body Fluids Precautions'** as outlined in Table 6.2.

Table 6.2 Blood/body fluid precautions

---

(1) Hands must be washed before and after nursing care.

(2) Gloves must be worn when handling blood, urine, faeces, secretions, or dealing with open wounds.

(3) Special care is required when handling needles and other sharps. Needles must not be bent or recapped after use, and must be discarded immediately in a puncture resistant, waterproof container.

(4) All specimens sent to the laboratory must be clearly labelled and placed in an impervious bag for transport. Appropriate labels include:
   - 'Risk of Infection'
   - 'Biohazard'
   - 'Blood/Body Fluid Precautions'

Labelling a specimen with 'AIDS precautions' is *not* necessary; any of the above is sufficient and is less likely to lead to a violation of the confidentiality of the patient's diagnosis.

Both the specimen and specimen request form must be similarly labelled.

(5) Spillages of blood and other body fluids must be saturated with an appropriate disinfectant (as previously discussed), left for 30 minutes, if possible, then carefully wiped up (by nursing personnel, *not* domestic or housekeeping staff) using disposable paper towels, which are then placed in the appropriate coloured plastic bag, and sent for incineration.

Ward accommodation: Because AIDS is a bloodborne, sexually transmitted disease, the *automatic* accommodation of patients with this disease in a single (private) room is not necessary. Quite clearly, with the
large number of individuals in the community currently infected with
this virus, hospitals will not have single room accommodation for all
patients who have AIDS or ARC, let alone for all patients who may be
sero-positive for anti-HIV. There is no reason why patients with AIDS
and HIV-related conditions cannot be nursed on an open ward with
complete safety. The nursing assessment of each patient will dictate
whether or not a single room is required. Table 6.3 summarizes the
indications when a single room is useful. As many patients with AIDS
will have nursing care issues outlined there, it is clear that a single room
will frequently be required. However, there is a difference between a
patient admitted with Kaposi's sarcoma for a biopsy (who does not
require a single room) and a seriously ill patient admitted with a host of
opportunistic infections. Patients not admitted to single rooms can
move about freely on the ward and other than for 'Blood/Body Fluid
Precautions,' do not require any restrictions. The major disadvantage
of admitting a patient into a single room is the further sense of isolation
and rejection felt by most patients with HIV-related conditions. As is
usual, all nursing care must be planned with the patient. Careful
explanation of IC precautions must be given to the patient. If a patient
is admitted to a single room, this does not necessarily mean that the
patient is *confined* to that room. For example, patients with diarrhoea
may be allowed full ward activities as appropriate.

All patients in single room accommodation must be frequently re-
assessed. The plan of care for each shift must allow time for nurses to
talk to patients, rather than just entering the room when there is something to do. Efforts must be made to ensure that domestic and catering
staff are aware of the IC precautions (*not* the diagnosis!), that meals are
delivered and the room cleaned. The final responsibility for the
patient's environment is a nursing responsibility.

Protective clothing – When a patient is admitted to a single room,
health care workers do *not* need to wear *any* protective clothing when
entering the room just to talk to the patient, deliver meals, post, newspapers, etc. Protective clothing is used in the following situations:
1. *Giving direct nursing care*: when entering a room to deliver direct
nursing care such as assisting a patient to bathe, dealing with bed-pans,
urinals or specimens, recording routine observations, changing dressings or dealing with incontinence, the *only* protective clothing necessary
is a disposable plastic apron and a pair of disposable gloves.

Table 6.3 Indications for single room accommodation

(1) Patients who have an opportunistic infection which normally requires a single room (e.g. pulmonary tuberculosis or salmonella infection).

(2) Patients who are bleeding, likely to bleed (e.g. thrombocytopenia, candida oesophagitis) or who have open or draining wounds.

(3) Grossly incontinent patients or those with severe diarrhoea.

(4) Neurological manifestations of HIV infection (e.g. confusion) which make it difficult for the patient to co-operate and maintain good standards of hygiene.

(5) Patients with conditions associated with excessive, productive coughing.

(6) Seriously ill patients who require high dependency nursing care.

(7) Terminally ill patients.

(8) Psychological or social reasons.

Gowns are *not* usually required, unless the patient is grossly incontinent. Gowns are not waterproof and, in most situations, do not offer any additional protection. Additional protective clothing is sometimes indicated, such as when dealing with spillages, assisting with invasive procedures (e.g. bronchoscopy), or managing a patient care situation in which there is likely to be a gross environmental contamination with blood or body fluids (e.g. a patient with haematemesis) or extensive draining wounds. In these circumstances, the following protective clothing is indicated: a plastic apron worn under a long-sleeved gown; a pair of disposable gloves; a mask and eye protection.

Most patients with HIV infection are also excretors of CMV and a mask and eye protection are appropriate in caring for patients who are coughing excessively, although the ability of patients to excrete significant amounts of CMV by coughing is not known. Some patients with AIDS have pulmonary tuberculosis and, in this condition, a mask is required. It may be more appropriate for *the patient* to wear a mask, for instance, when being transported to another department for investigations or treatment, in which case it is unnecessary for health care workers to do so also.

Appropriate disposable gloves are usually those made out of rubber latex, *not* plastic examination gloves. Suitable face masks are high filtration types used in surgery, not flimsy, tissue thin paper masks. Eye protection devices should not resemble underwater goggles. Simple plastic or normal-looking glasses with plain glass lenses are available. If health care workers already wear glasses, they do not need to wear additional eye protection. In general, if a face mask is required, eye protection should be worn.

Catering staff do not need to wear any protective clothing to deliver meals. Housekeeping and domestic staff need only wear a plastic apron and a pair of disposable gloves when cleaning the room. Physiotherapists should wear gloves, plastic apron and a face mask when giving chest physiotherapy. Social workers and other members of the hospital staff need not wear any protective clothing. Medical staff follow the same IC guidelines as those described for nursing personnel.

In general, visitors require no protective clothing, unless they are assisting in patient care activities with nursing personnel, who will advise them appropriately.

In patients who have pulmonary involvement, the nurse in charge will be able to advise other health care workers and visitors when a face mask is required.

As pneumonia caused by *P. carinii* is one of the most common opportunistic diseases seen in patients with AIDS, it is worth stressing that this particular condition is not infectious to health care workers and others who have a normal immune response.

Injections and sharps: Probably the *only* time the nurse faces a significant potential risk of infection with HIV is when giving injections, caring for intravenous infusion sites or dealing with blood-contaminated sharp instruments, *especially needles*. Disposable syringes and needles must be used and gloves are worn when giving injections or caring for infusion sites and when handling any contaminated sharp instruments. Needle-locking syringes or one-piece needle-syringe units should be used. In general, student nurses should not give injections to patients who have a blood-borne infectious disease; injections should only be given by Registered Nurses.

Needles must not be reinserted into their original sheaths or bent after use. It is generally unnecessary to detach the needle from the syringe after use and needles and syringes should be promptly discarded as one unit, into a rigid, puncture-proof plastic container, which is kept by (or taken to) the patient's bedside. When the 'sharps container' is three quarters full, it is sealed, labelled appropriately (e.g. 'Risk of Infection' or 'BioHazard') and sent for incineration. The one exception is that when either venesectionists or medical staff take blood, they must remove the needle from the syringe before ejecting it into the specimen container to prevent a microscopic aerosol spray.

Bed pans and urinals: most patients will be able to use toilet facilities in their room. It is not necessary to pour disinfectants into the toilet after use; routine cleaning by housekeeping or domestic staff (wearing gloves!) is all that is required. If bed pans or urinals are used, they should be emptied as per the usual ward procedure by nursing staff (wearing plastic aprons and gloves). Disposable bed pans and urinals that require crushing for disposal (e.g. paper mâché equipment) should not be used. Clearly each patient requires his own individual bed pan and urinal, which may be emptied into the patient's toilet, taking care not to splash the contents, and then rinsed. It is not necessary to soak the bedpan or urinal after use in any disinfectant. They should be stored dry in the patient's room. Bedpans and urinals may also be emptied into a 'bedpan washer,' making sure that the door is securely closed before turning on the machine. Many patients with AIDS will have profuse diarrhoea and if they are not able to use their own toilet, a bedside commode is preferable to using a bedpan in bed.

Linen: contaminated linen is double-bagged. It is first placed in a *red*, plastic bag (preferably an 'alginate – stitched' or polyvinyl alcohol bag), which is then placed into a *red* nylon bag. In the National Health Service (UK), all linen placed in *red*, nylon bags is infected linen, and no other labelling is required. Hospital laundries have their own procedure for dealing with infected linen, which, since the virus responsible is sensitive to heat and detergents, is usually washed separately in hot, soapy water. Many times, a disinfectant, such as hypochlorite, is added. If linen is *grossly* contaminated with blood or other body fluids, it may be the hospital's procedure to send it for incineration, rather than for processing in the laundry.

Rubbish: used dressings, paper towels, tubing, and other rubbish is placed in a heavy duty, plastic bag, sealed, and sent for incineration. In the National Health Service (UK), contaminated rubbish placed in *yellow* plastic bags is always incinerated. Additional labelling is not required. When disposing of intravenous tubing, great care must be taken by nursing personnel to ensure that needles and other sharps have first been removed. This may require careful cutting off of *both* sharp ends. Patients who are not in a single room, may dispose of their rubbish (e.g. newspapers, etc.) in the ordinary way, as long as it is not contaminated by blood or other body fluids. In the National Health Service (UK), non-infectious rubbish is disposed of in *black* plastic bags.

Crockery and cutlery: patients with HIV infection do not generally require disposable crockery and cutlery. In those situations where the patient has a severe mouth infection, pulmonary tuberculosis, or an enteric infection, it is preferable that they use their own normal crockery and cutlery, which can be kept in the patient's room. Often the patient, or the patient's visitors, can assist in washing these few dishes and silver or it can be done by nursing personnel. Rarely are disposable crockery and cutlery needed.

Instruments: used instruments should be placed in a plastic bag or a special plastic box before being returned to the Central Sterile Supply Department (CSSD) for re-sterilizing. Instruments which cannot be autoclaved (e.g. endoscopic instruments), should be placed in glutaraldehyde 2% for one hour, washed with a detergent and warm water and left in glutaraldehyde 2% for three hours, then rinsed and stored dried. Although HIV can be easily inactivated by most disinfectants, as patients with AIDS frequently have several opportunistic infections, disinfectants which are mycobacteriocidal are used for disinfecting all instruments which cannot be autoclaved. The hospital's specific procedure for using these disinfectants (or the manufacturer's instructions) must be meticulously followed. The advice of the Control of Infection Nurse should be sought if there is any confusion about how these agents should be used.

Contaminated surfaces: surfaces which may have been contaminated during procedures (e.g. dressing trolleys, tables, and bench surfaces), should be wiped with a *weak* solution of hypochlorite (1000 ppm of available chlorine – i.e. household bleach diluted 1 part bleach to 100 parts of water) or freshly prepared glutaraldehyde 2% (NB hypochlorite is corrosive to metal surfaces and fabrics). Grossly contaminated surfaces should be cleaned with either glutaraldehyde 2% or a *strong* solution of hypochlorite (10 000 ppm – a 1 in 10 dilution of household bleach) which should, where possible, be left in contact with the contaminated surface for 30 minutes, prior to being wiped up with disposable paper towels.

Handwashing: Hands must be washed before and after all patient contact, thus avoiding the introduction of new potential pathogens to an already immunocompromised patient and to prevent transmitting opportunistic microorganisms to other patients. Iodophors (complexes of iodine and solubilizers) such as povidone-iodine ('Betadine', 'Videne') are appropriate as these halogenated soaps have been shown to eradicate HIV[12], and are effective against a wide range of potential pathogens. The use of gloves does not eliminate the need for good handwashing techniques.

Table 6.4 summarizes the standard IC precautions that are used with patients who have fully expressed AIDS or ARC. When a patient is admitted, after a nursing history is taken and the original patient care assessment is completed, the nurse may make out an **IC Precautions Card** (as shown in Figure 6.1), adapting the above general IC Guidelines for the individual patient. All patients with AIDS are not the same. It is not appropriate to have a rigid procedure for AIDS patients, which is implemented without modification each time a patient with this condition is admitted.

Table 6.4 Standard IC precautions – AIDS and ARC

Precaution	Procedure	Rationale
1. Single room	Used for patients with severe diarrhoea, excessive coughing, some opportunistic infections, seriously or terminally ill, bleeding or anticipated bleeding, enteric infections, or for psychological or social reasons.	To protect the immunocompromised patient from nosocomial infections, and to protect health care workers and other patients from infection with HIV and associated opportunistic pathogens.
2. Plastic aprons and gloves	Used when delivering direct patient care, handling specimens, or domestic cleaning.	As above.

continued

Table 6.4   *Cont'd*

Precaution	Procedure	Rationale
3. Gowns, masks and eye protection. NB: A plastic apron is always worn underneath a gown.	Only used in dealing with gross contamination or assisting with invasive procedures, or when the patient is coughing excessively, or at any time in which aerosol contamination is anticipated. Masks without eye protection, either worn by the patient outside the room, or by health care workers inside the room, are required during the early treatment phase for patients with pulmonary tuberculosis.	To protect health care workers from infection with HIV or other associated opportunistic pathogens (e.g., *Mycobacterium tuberculosis*, CMV). To protect health care workers from acquisition of *M. tuberculosis* infection.
4. Handwashing	Hands are washed prior to, and after all patient care activities. If gloves are worn, hands must still be carefully washed prior to gloving, and after gloves are removed. Povidone–iodine 7.5% in a non–ionic detergent base ('Betadine' or 'Videne' Surgical Scrub) is preferred.	To protect the immunocompromised patient from nosocomial infection and to protect health care workers from aquisition of HIV and associated opportunistic pathogens. To prevent transmission of potential pathogens to other patients.

Table 6.4 *Cont'd*

Precaution	Procedure	Rationale
5. Needles, injections, and other sharps	Injections given by Registered Nurses only. Needles are not re-capped, bent, or broken after use and are disposed of immediately in a rigid, plastic, puncture-resistant and waterproof 'Sharps container'. Sharps container is taken to bedside or left in patient's room. Special care is required for disposing of intravenous infusion sets. Used instruments are placed in waterproof plastic bag or plastic box and returned to CSSD for autoclaving.	Meticulous care is required in dealing with sharps to prevent needle-stick injuries with possible HIV acquisition by health care workers. Needles are not broken or snapped off in order to avoid a microscopic aerosol of infected material. If sharp ends not carefully cut off there is a risk that they will puncture side of plastic disposal bags, and injure ancillary staff. To prevent leakage of blood or body fluids while being transported to the CSSD.
6. Linen	Double-bagged. First placed in red, plastic alginate bag, which in turn is placed in a red, nylon bag, and then closed securely and sent to the laundry. Gloves are worn when making beds and handling infected linen.	To prevent contamination of housekeeping personnel when transporting linen to laundry, and to protect laundry personnel from contamination by infected linen.

continued

Table 6.4 *Cont'd*

Precaution	Procedure	Rationale
7. Contaminated material	All infected rubbish, including dressings, drainage tubing and intravenous fluid administration sets (with sharp ends cut off at both ends!) are placed in a heavy-duty yellow plastic bag, securely closed, and sent for incineration.	To protect housekeeping and portering personnel from contamination. Scrupulous care must be taken to ensure no sharps are placed in rubbish bags.
8. Crockery and cutlery	May use ordinary dishes and silverware. If patient has an enteric or mouth infection, or has pulmonary tuberculosis, may keep individual dishes and silver in room.	Disposable crockery and cutlery rarely needed. To prevent risk of transmitting opportunistic pathogens to other patients.
9. Specimens	Gloves are worn when handling all specimens. Specimen container and specimen request form are labelled with a suitable warning sticker (e.g. 'BioHazard' or 'Risk of Infection') and transported to the laboratory in an impervious plastic bag.	To prevent contamination with infected blood and body fluids, affecting everyone who is handling specimens. To alert laboratory personnel of special risk. To prevent leakage during transport to laboratory.
10. Ward privileges and visitors	If ambulatory, may have full ward privileges (e.g. may go to TV room, Hospital Shop, etc.)	To prevent isolation.

Table 6.4 *Cont'd*

Precaution	Procedure	Rationale
	Patients with diarrhoea should use their own toilet.	To prevent contamination.
	Visitors are to be encouraged.	

Needless to say, patients admitted to hospital for assessment who do not have fully expressed AIDS, but have ARC or are seropositive for anti-HIV, do not require extensive IC precautions. They only require 'Blood/Body Fluids Precautions,' as described in Table 6.2.

It is essential that medical staff inform nursing personnel when a patient is admitted, either with AIDS or ARC, or who is known to be seropositive for anti-HIV, or who is being investigated for these conditions. This will allow sensible IC precautions to be incorporated in the nursing care plan.

Because of the vast numbers of individuals in the community who are currently infected with this retrovirus and are unaware of it, nurses will often be caring for patients in which the infection is unidentified. Therefore it is logical to adopt sensible IC procedures for *all* patients. Special care must now be taken to avoid contamination with blood and body fluids from *every* patient. Strict attention must be paid to good handwashing techniques, wearing gloves when dealing with *all* blood and body fluids. Diligent care when dealing with needles and other sharps has now become even more obligatory in nursing care. With the advent of AIDS, the days of nurses adopting a casual approach to blood and body fluids from any patient are gone forever. If a nurse or other health care worker has a parenteral (e.g., needlestick or cut) or mucous membrane (e.g. splash to the eye or mouth) exposure to blood or other body fluids, the instructions in Table 6.5 should be followed.

Table 6.5 Procedure for treating parenteral or mucous membrane exposure to blood/body fluids

1. *Parenteral exposure*:
   - injury should be encouraged to bleed by local venous occlusion
   - this is followed by washing the inoculation site for 5 minutes in running water, using povidone–iodine 7.5% in a detergent base ('Betadine' or 'Videne' surgical scrub), or other suitable antiseptic solution, or soap.

continued

Table 6.5   *Cont'd*

2. *Mucous membrane exposure*:
    - splashes in the mouth: the mouth should be washed out, using running water
    - splashes into the eye: the eye should be well irrigated with either running water or sodium chloride 0.9%.

3. The accident should immediately be reported to the senior nurse in charge and an 'Incident Report' should be made out, fully documenting the accident.

4. The nurse should be seen in the Occupational Health Department, or by his/her own physician, who will advise on serological screening for anti-HIV.

5. *Serological screening for anti-HIV*: A base-line specimen of blood should be taken immediately and either tested for anti-HIV, or stored frozen. Further specimens of blood are not required unless there is a clinical indication for them. If the nurse wishes, serological follow-up can be offered, however possible implications of a positive result must be clearly discussed.

6. The nurse should be examined and health status documented every six months for one year following the accident. This also provides an opportunity to offer reassurance.

Nurses or other health care workers who have cuts, abrasions or any type of skin lesion, should ensure that these are covered with a waterproof dressing, and that gloves are worn when caring for any patient in whom it is anticipated that exposure to blood or other body fluids may occur. This is even more crucial when caring for patients with AIDS or ARC or who are known to be anti-HIV positive.

It is reassuring, however, that to date, no nursing personnel have contracted AIDS from caring for patients infected with HIV. Despite hundreds of needle-stick injuries among nurses and doctors associated with caring for a patient with AIDS, less than six have even seroconverted. In the United States, a nationwide prospective surveillance of health care workers with documented parenteral or mucous membrane exposures to blood or other body fluids of patients with AIDS or ARC involved 938 health care workers who were followed serologically after exposure. Most exposures (76%) were a result of needlestick injuries or cuts with contaminated sharp instruments, the vast majority (>85%)

being exposed to blood or serum. Only two health care workers sero-converted[13]. A summary of further studies[14] has confirmed the low infectivity of HTLV-III in a health care setting. Despite the fact that most needlestick injuries do not seem to transmit the infection, nurses and other health care workers must be extremely vigilant in guarding against this potentially catastrophic accident. It is sad to note that the first case of a nurse who did seroconvert following a severe needlestick injury occurred in England[15].

References

1. Spire, B., Barre–Sinoussi, F., Montagnier, L., *et al.* (1985). Inactivation of lymphadenopathy-associated virus by heat, Gamma rays, and ultraviolet light. *Lancet.* (26 January) i(8422):188–9

2. DHSS (1986). Acquired Immune Deficiency Syndrome (AIDS) Booklet 3 – Guidance for Surgeons, Anaesthetists, Dentists and their Teams in Dealing with Patients infected with HTLV-III (April). CMO(86)7

3. Grouse, L.D. (1985). HTLV-III transmission. *Journal of the American Medical Association.* (18 October) 254:2130-1

4. Spire, B., Montagnier, L., Barre–Sinoussi, F., and Chermann, J.C. (1984). Inactivation of lymphadenopathy associated virus by chemical disinfectants. *Lancet* (20 October) ii(8408):899–901

5. DHSS and the Health & Safety Executive (1984). Advisory Committee on Dangerous Pathogens (ACDP). Acquired Immune Deficiency Syndrome (AIDS) – Interim Guidelines (December)

6. Centers for Disease Control (CDC) (1986). Recommended infection-control practices for dentistry. *MMWR* (18 April) 35(15):237–242

7. Centers for Disease Control (CDC) (1985) Summary: Recommendations for preventing transmission of infection with human T-lymphotropic virus type III/lymphadenopathy-associated virus in the work place. *MMWR* (15 November) 34(45):681–695

8. *Ibid.*

9. DHSS and the Health & Safety Executive (ACDP) (1984). *loc. cit.*

10. DHSS (1986) *loc. cit.*

11. Royal College of Nursing. London. (1985, updated 1986). Nursing Guidelines on the Management of Patients in Hospital and the Community suffering from AIDS

12. Martin, L.S., McDougal, S., Loskoski, S.L. (1985). Disinfection and inactivation of the human T-lymphotropic virus type III/lymphadenopathy-associated virus. *Journal of Infectious Diseases* 152:400–03

13. McCray, E. (The Cooperative Needlestick Surveillance Group). (1986). Special Report: Occupational risk of the Acquired Immunodeficiency Syndrome among health care workers. *The New England Journal of Medicine.* (24 April) 314(17):1127-32

14. Geddes, A.M. (1986). Risk of AIDS to health care workers. *British Medical Journal* (15 March) 292(6522):711–12

15. Anonymous (1984). Needlestick transmission of HTLV3 from a patient infected in Africa [editorial]. *Lancet* (15 December) ii(8416):1376-7

7

The Individualized Care of Patients with AIDS

Strategic nursing care embraces the concept of a problem-solving approach to the individualized care of each patient. However, it is more than a nursing process style of care. It includes assessment and planning of nursing care on a hospital-wide basis, taking into consideration all the real and possible issues governing the implementation of care and includes both logistical, educational and managerial aspects, which, if not anticipated, may preclude the delivery of individualized, high quality care. In this chapter we are going to explore planned care for individual patients; further chapters will discuss the issues and back-up nursing support required to deliver this care effectively.

Strategic nursing care: a model for patients with HIV-related disease

Behavioural models of nursing, as conceived by Henderson[1], Roper[2] and Orem[3], are valuable tools by which individualized nursing care of patients with HIV-related disease can be planned and implemented efficiently and effectively. These models describe needs and self-care requisites necessary for normal, healthy living. The use of these models allows for the speedy identification by the nurse of unmet needs and deficits in self-care requisites. A nursing assessment includes the recognition of unmet needs and actual problems. It further identifies potential problems associated with the patient's condition (social, psychological, physical and medical), specific illness, hospitalization and medical treatment. Identifying and documenting needs, self-care requisites, actual problems and potential problems facilitates planning appropriate nursing intervention and allows the effectiveness of this intervention to be evaluated. In discussing the strategic nursing care of patients with HIV-related disease, an eclectic approach to behavioural models of nursing has been used. The overall objective of planned nursing care is to 'assist the individual, sick or well, in the performance of those activities contributing to health or its recovery (or to peaceful death) that he would perform unaided if he had the necessary strength, will or knowledge. And to do this in such a way as to help him gain independence as rapidly as possible'[4].

Needs

In common with all individuals, patients with HIV-related disease have needs which they or others must meet for health to be maintained. Table 7.1, adapted from Henderson's *Components of basic nursing*[5] and Roper's *Activities of Living*[6] lists the needs which may be examined during the nursing assessment.

Table 7.1 Requisites for health

1. The need for adequate respiration
2. The need for adequate hydration
3. The need for adequate nutrition
4. The need for urinary and faecal elimination
5. The need to control body temperature
6. The need for movement and mobilisation
7. The need for a safe environment
8. The need for personal cleansing and dressing
9. The need for expression and communication
10. The need for working and playing
11. The need for adequate rest and sleep
12. The need to maintain psychological equilibrium
13. The need to worship according to his own faith
14. The need to express sexuality
15. Needs associated with dying

By examining these requisites or needs, problems may be identified. These may be either current problems (Actual Problems) or problems that may be anticipated due to the patient's need deprivation, medical condition or treatment (Potential Problems).

1. The need for adequate respiration

Potential problems
1.1 dyspnoea, cough, tachypnoea, cyanosis

Origin of problem
pneumonia (*P. carinii*, CMV other opportunistic pathogen) neoplastic involvement from Kaposi's sarcoma or anaemia

Objectives of care
1. To maintain optimal respiratory function
2. To alleviate cough
3. To keep patient well oxygenated

Nursing intervention

Assessment: Vital signs (blood pressure/pulse/respiratory rate), arterial blood gases (ABG), colour, respiratory effort, chest sounds, sputum production and mental status should be noted and documented as a base-line assessment.

Position: The patient should be placed in a position which facilitates good respiratory function. Sitting the patient upright, leaning forward and well supported is frequently useful in that it allows the accessory muscles (sternomastoid, pectoralis major, platysma and latissimus dorsi) to assist respiratory effort.

Oxygen: Depending on the patient's clinical condition and arterial blood gases (ABG), the physician may prescribe supplemental oxygen to be administered. In general, the lowest concentration of oxygen needed to overcome hypoxaemia will be ordered. Concentrations of inspired oxygen < 40 per cent are well tolerated for long periods of time and may be administered by Ventimasks (Vickers Limited Medical Group) or Edinburgh masks (British Oxygen Co. Ltd.). Double nasal cannulae may be preferred as they are comfortable and do not interfere with eating, drinking and the wearing of spectacles, although the inspired oxygen concentration provided is unpredictable. An oxygen flow rate of 2 litres/minute will provide approximately a 30 per cent concentration. High concentrations of supplemental oxygen are sometimes required. They can be administered by Polymasks (British Oxygen Co. Ltd.) or MC masks (Medical and Industrial Equipment Ltd.), both of which deliver approximately a 60 per cent concentration at a flow rate of 4–6 litres/minute. Oxygen administered by these masks requires humidification. Oxygen concentrations of > 60 per cent, which have significant toxic effects on the alveolar capillary endothelium and bronchi should not be used for long periods unless absolutely necessary for the patient's survival. Oxygen therapy should be continuous rather than intermittent, aiming to maintain a constant arterial partial pressure of oxygen (aPO2) between 60–80 mm Hg.

Patient education: Patients should be taught deep breathing and coughing exercises. The employment of an incentive spirometer is useful for deep breathing exercises.

Chest physiotherapy: Extensive chest physiotherapy will be required to assist in establishing and maintaining clear lung fields.

Suction: Patients with severe respiratory embarrassment will require suction. Disposable gloves, plastic apron, high filtration mask and eye protection are necessary when suctioning patients as explosive coughing releases a potentially contaminated aerosol spray.

Medications: Medications are administered as prescribed and potential side effects should be anticipated. These include:

Medication	Possible side effects
pentamidine isethionate	hypoglycaemia (or more rarely, hyperglycaemia)
	hypotension
NB: test urine twice daily for	abscesses at injection
sugar and acetone.	sites – skin rashes
Monitor daily	tachycardia
blood glucose	pruritus
estimates (normal:	thrombocytopenia
2.5 – 4.7 mmol/l)	
(45–85 mg/100 ml)	
trimethoprim-	drug fever
sulfamethoxazole	rash
(co-trimoxazole)	leukopenia
Others: DFMO (difluoro-	nausea and vomiting; various
methylomithine), sulfadoxine	haematological disorders – rash
and pyrimethamine & Dapsone	nephrotoxicity; neurological
	disorders

Other medications may be prescribed including **expectorants** (bromhexine HCL or mixtures containing either syrup of ipecac, guaifensin or saturated solution of potassium iodide), **cough suppressants** (mixtures containing either dextromethorphan, codeine phosphate or pholcodine), and other **antibiotics**.

Reassurance: Patients with respiratory distress require frequent reassurance from the nurse. They are often anxious, tending to panic if they feel they cannot breathe. The 'nurse call system' should be placed within easy reach of the patient.

Mouth care: Oxygen is drying to mucous membranes and frequent mouth care will be required. Patients should rinse their mouth out with water or a pleasantly flavoured mouthwash solution every hour.

Nasal care: If nasal cannulae are used, it is useful if the anterior nares are lightly coated with a protective ointment, such as vaseline or glycerine.

Evaluation: Patients should be re-assessed frequently and changes in

- vital signs and body temperature
- colour
- sputum production
- chest sounds
- arterial blood gases

documented. Changes in respiratory status must be reported to the physician immediately. The patient must also be frequently re-assessed for signs of new chest infections. Frequent measurements of arterial blood pressure must be made while patients are receiving pentamidine isethionate.

2.   The need for adequate hydration

Potential problems   **Origin of problem**
2.1   Dehydration   *Inadequate intake of oral fluids*:
                               dysphagia secondary to *Candida
                               albicans* infection or KS lesions
                               lethargy, confusion or coma

                               Fluid loss: diarrhoea, nausea,
                               vomiting, GI suctioning
                               fever and diaphoresis
                               hyperpnoea

2.2   Electrolyte imbalance   diarrhoea, nausea, vomiting, GI
                               suctioning

Objectives of care
1.   To correct dehydration and electrolyte imbalance
2.   To maintain optimal hydration and electrolyte homeostasis

Nursing intervention

Assessment: The patient should be weighed daily (at the same time each day) and an exact record of fluid intake and output maintained. Skin turgor should be assessed on a daily basis.

Oral fluids: The patient should be encouraged to drink frequent, small amounts of oral fluids as tolerated. For all patients, especially those with fever, a plentiful supply of fresh iced water should be kept on the patient's bedside locker.

Intravenous rehydration: The physician will prescribe a regime of intravenous fluids. These fluids must be infused at the correct flow rate, as ordered by the physician.

Electrolyte replacement: Electrolytes will be added to intravenous infusions according to the physician's prescription. Patients with potassium imbalance may be continuously assessed by using a cardiac monitor.

Mouth care: Dehydrated patients require frequent (2 hourly) mouth care.

Evaluation: Effective rehydration and electrolyte replacement will result in normal skin turgor, blood pressure, heart rate and absence of signs of mental confusion or vertigo (if due to dehydration).

Plasma electrolyte levels should be carefully monitored and results outside normal parameters reported to the physician immediately.

Normal electrolyte parameters:

Potassium:	3.8 – 5.0 mmol/l	(mEq/l)
sodium:	135 – 145 mmol/l	(mEq/l)
chloride:	100 – 106 mmol/l	(mEq/l)

3. The need for adequate nutrition

Actual problem	Origin of problem
3.1 weight loss	catabolism associated with AIDS

Potential problems	
3.2 further severe weight loss and malnutrition	increased catabolism, fever, diarrhoea, nausea and vomiting profound anorexia dysphagia – KS lesions in GI tract, malabsorption

Objectives of care
1. To keep patient well nourished
2. To prevent further weight loss
3. To enhance weight gain

Nursing intervention

Assessment: Weigh patient and take history of previous dietary patterns, including likes, dislikes and any known food allergies. Note the current dietary habit of the patient as many patients with AIDS will be on special diets, often as 'alternative' forms of treatment (e.g. macrobiotic diets). The dietitian should be informed of the patient's admission and, after interviewing the patient, will be able to advise on a nutritional regime.

Oral nutrition: The patient may tolerate small, frequent meals better than the traditional three meals a day. Every effort should be made to present the patient with food he likes. This can be brought in by visitors if it is not readily available in the hospital. Yogurts and meal substitutes ('Carnation,' 'Ensure Plus') are often well tolerated. If allowed by the physician, a small amount of sherry prior to meals may stimulate appetite. Prescribed anti-emetics should be given an hour before meals. Usually the dietitian will advise the physician on any special diets ordered for the patient. Some patients may wish to follow their own special diet, such as a macrobiotic diet. This may present a conflict as current medical opinion does not feel this diet is useful in a catabolic condition. This can be discussed with the patient but, in the end, his wishes must be respected. He may feel his diet is his only remaining hope.

Enteral tube feeding: Enteral feeding is often employed in AIDS patients who are seriously ill and cannot be maintained on oral nutrition. A naso–gastric tube is passed, usually being left *in situ*. Isotonic, lactose-free formulae are often employed, the solution generally being administered at between 50–100 ml an hour, depending on the patient's tolerance of it. Diarrhoea is a severe reaction to enteral feeding but may be controlled by reducing the rate of administration. An alternative regime is to pass a naso–gastric tube, leaving it *in situ* for a morning or an afternoon and only feeding the patient during this time, making up nutritional requirements with either oral or parenteral feeds.

Parenteral nutrition: Solutions of protein, lipids and carbohydrates may be infused intravenously. Trace elements, electrolytes and vitamins may be added. Short-term peripheral parenteral nutrition can be employed, although it is more usual for parenteral nutrition to be administered via a central line. There are risks associated with total parenteral nutrition (TPN). Patients frequently become hyperglycaemic due to the carbohydrate load. Insulin may be added to the solution to control this. All patients on TPN should have four hourly urinalysis for sugar and ketone bodies as well as daily blood glucose estimates. Great care must be taken of the infusion site and line as they frequently become infected. When TPN is discontinued, it must be done *gradually* and the patient carefully observed for signs of hypoglycaemia.

Medications: *Anti-emetics* are almost universally prescribed for patients with AIDS who have nausea and vomiting. Probably the most frequently used anti-emetic is metoclopramide ('Maxolon'), which can be given either orally or by intramuscular or intravenous injection. Anti-emetic suppositories such as thiethylperazine maleate ('Torecan') may be useful with some patients. *Antidiarrhoeals* may be effective with some patients. However they are notoriously ineffective in many patients with AIDS who have severe diarrhoea. The most common anti-diarrhoeals used include diphenoxylate HCL with atropine sulphate ('Lomotil') and loperamide HCL ('Imodium'). Codeine phosphate may also be used. *Supplemental vitamins*: Most patients with AIDS will have vitamin supplements prescribed. Many will be on their own regime of 'mega-dose' vitamin therapy. As fat-soluble vitamins (A,D,E and K) are toxic in high doses, the physician must be aware of any medication the patient has brought in with him and is taking in hospital. This includes vitamin preparations.

Evaluation: If nutritional support is successful, the patient should show a weight gain or, at least, a cessation of weight loss. Unfortunately, weight loss and malnutrition are generally profound, persistent and progressive. The patient must be weighed daily (at the same time each day) and recordings of fluid intake and output maintained. Abdominal girth is measured daily (again, at the same time each day). The patient's abdomen is marked clearly so that all nursing personnel measure the girth consistently. Bowel sounds should be assessed four hourly when on enteral feeding.

4.   The need for urinary and faecal elimination

Potential problems	Origin of problems
4.1 diarrhoea	Opportunistic infections (e.g., cryptosporidiosis, CMV amoebiasis, *Isospora belli*), KS lesions in the GI tract, or of idiopathic origin
oliguria	dehydration
incontinence	confusion, loss of mobility, terminal illness

Objectives of care
1. To control or minimize effects of diarrhoea and incontinence
2. To achieve effective implementation of enteric IC precautions, if indicated
3. To facilitate correction of water imbalance

Nursing intervention

Assessment: Frequency of bowel movements should be documented and fluid intake and output recorded.

Toilet facilities: Patients with diarrhoea should be nursed in a single room which has private toilet facilities. If the patient is not ambulatory, a bedside commode is preferable to using a bedpan in bed. Bedpans may be carefully emptied (to avoid splashing) in the patient's toilet, or the contents disposed of in the bedpan washer.

Skin care: The skin must be kept clean and dry. It is essential that facilities are made available for the patient to wash his hands after using the toilet. If the patient is incontinent, protective or barrier creams may be useful in preventing excoriation of the skin (e.g. 'Sprilon' spray – Pharmacia GB Ltd., or 'Vitamin A + D Ointment – Emollient' – E. Fougera & Co.).

Hydration: Patients with severe diarrhoea may become quickly dehydrated and the patient must be encouraged to drink adequate amounts of fluids to replace those lost due to diarrhoea. Intravenous rehydration may be necessary in some patients.

Nursing care of the incontinent patient: Urinary incontinence may be managed by leaving an urinal carefully placed between the patient's legs. Alternatively, external catheters, such as the 'Texas' latex penile sheath (Cory Bros. Ltd.) or 'Uro-Flow' non-allergenic penile sheaths, with hypo-allergenic, adhesive, distensible foam liners (Downs Surgical Ltd.) may be used. Patients with faecal incontinence should be nursed on clean, dry incontinent pads, which are placed on a linen drawsheet over a plastic sheet. All patients who are incontinent must be checked hourly.

Diet: The dietitian may be consulted in order to assess if a change in the patient's diet may assist in controlling faecal incontinence.

Pressure area care: Patients who are incontinent, are at an increased risk of developing pressure sores. Pressure area care, including turning the patient on alternative sides, should be undertaken every two hours. It is useful to re-assess the patient daily using the Norton scale[7].

Infection control: Nurses must wear rubber or latex disposable gloves (of the correct size!) and plastic aprons when disposing of urine or faeces and when caring for incontinent patients. Contaminated linen is double-bagged in a red, plastic bag, which is then placed in a red, nylon bag, sealed and sent to the laundry. Careful handwashing, prior to and after caring for patients is exceptionally important with patients who have enteric infections. Wearing gloves does not decrease the need for good handwashing technique. If patients have enteric infections, they should have their own set of crockery and cutlery, which may be kept in the patient's room. This can be washed by the nurse after use. This is preferable to presenting food to a patient with gastro–intestinal symptoms on unattractive disposable paper plates and asking him to use plastic knives, spoons and forks.

Evaluation: Effective nursing intervention will prevent dehydration secondary to severe diarrhoea, skin excoriation and pressure area breakdown. It will also help to minimize the psychological effects of severe diarrhoea and/or incontinence.

5. The need to control body temperature

Potential problem   **Origin of problem**
5.1   Fever and night sweats   Opportunistic infections

Objectives of care
1.   To assist in maintaining normal body temperature (36 to 37.5 degrees C)
2.   To keep the patient comfortable

Nursing intervention

Assessment: Patients with AIDS and ARC should have vital signs and body temperature recorded four-hourly. The occurrence of night sweats is common in both conditions and should be documented in the nursing notes.

Medication: The physician may prescribe medication to reduce body temperature, such as aspirin or paracetamol BP (acetaminophen USP). These should be administered as ordered.

Comfort: The patient should be kept clean, dry and well hydrated. Prolonged fever increases metabolic processes. The patient should be encouraged to eat a nutritious diet. Glucose drinks, such as 'Lucozade' may be beneficial to some patients, although they may exacerbate diarrhoea in others. Bed clothes and linen should be light, dry and clean. If hyperpyrexia occurs, sponging with tepid water may prove useful. Iced drinks must be available for the patient with fever.

Evaluation: Pyrexia and intermittent fevers should be detected promptly and medication administered as per the physician's orders.

6.   The need for movement and mobilization

Potential problems	Origin of problem
6.1 muscle atrophy	restricted mobility
6.2 decubitus ulcers	weakness and bed
6.3 deep vein thrombosis	rest
	catabolism

Objectives of care
1. To prevent the formation of decubitus ulcers and deep vein thrombosis
2. To minimize muscle wasting
3. To achieve full mobilization and independence within the limits of the patient's abilities

Nursing intervention

Assessment: The patient's level of independence and ability to ambulate, along with any signs of muscle wasting, pressure sores or venous thrombosis will be assessed daily.

Physiotherapy: Patients not confined to bed should be walked frequently and encouraged to be as independent as possible. Patients on bed rest must have active and passive lower limb exercises and their position changed every two hours. A pull-rope, attached to the end of the bed, or a trapeze bar on a bed frame may prove useful with many patients.

Pressure area care: Patients on bed rest or semi bed rest must have two-hourly pressure area care. Gentle massage with a lanolin-based cream ('TLC' cream or Baby Lotion) is soothing to the patient and allows an opportunity for the nurse to inspect pressure sites. Patients with

restricted mobility should be commenced on a Norton scoring scale[8] as
illustrated in Figure 7.1.

Norton's scoring scale		
Patient's name:	Date:	

Physical condition:
Good 4
Fair 3
Poor 2 Score: _____
V. bad 1

Mental condition:
Alert 4
Apathetic 3
Confused 2 Score: _____
Stuporous 1

Activity:
Ambulant 4
Walk/help 3
Chairbound 2 Score: _____
Bedfast 1

Mobility:
Full 4
Sl. limited 3
V. limited 2 Score: _____
Immobile 1

Incontinent:
Not 4
Occasionally 3
Usually/ur. 2 Score: _____
Doubly 1

* * * Total score:

Fig. 7.1 Norton's scoring scale

Patients with a total score of 14 or less are prone to develop pressure
sores and patients with a total score below 12 are more likely than not to
develop pressure sores.

It is also useful to commence a patient on a 'Relief of pressure
chart'[9] as illustrated in Figure 7.2.

Nursing care must be organized in order to turn the patient every two
hours and lifting must be skilful in order to prevent shearing force to the
skin. The skin must be kept dry, cool and clean. Dehydration, malnutrition and anaemia are all predisposing factors to the development of
pressure sores. When possible, these must be corrected.

Evaluation: Effective nursing care will promote mobilization and independence and result in absence of pressure sores, venous thrombosis and excessive muscle wasting.

Relief of pressure chart				
Date	Time	Position of patient	Relief of pressure achieved by	Nurse's signature
12/11	0800	Lying on back	Turned on left side	W Jones.
"	1000	Lying on left side	Turned on right side	E. Karn
"	1200	Lying on right side	Turned on to back	J. baard.
"	1400	Lying on back	Turned on left side	A. Hilton

Fig. 7.2   Relief of pressure chart

7.   The need for a safe environment

Potential problems
7.1   nosocomial infection
7.2   accidents

Origin of problem
immunodeficiency
weakness
confusion
hospital environment and
equipment
CMV retinitis

Objectives of care
1.   To prevent nosocomial infection
2.   To maintain a safe environment

Nursing intervention

Assessment: An assessment of the patient's mental status includes determining his ability to understand and co-operate in his planned care. The patient's physical condition is assessed, including sight, a history of vertigo, seizures, falls and general state of debilitation.

Infection control: Infection control (IC) procedures will be implemented as per the previous chapter on this aspect of nursing care. All patients with immunodeficiency are at increased risk of nosocomial (i.e. hospital-acquired) infection, although patients with AIDS/ARC are more in danger of previously-acquired, latent infection. As patients with AIDS/ARC cannot protect themselves from new infections, it is essential that when in hospital they are not exposed to the added risk of nosocomial infections.

Safety: The following aspects must be taken into account when care is planned in order to maintain a safe environment:

1. *Oxygen*:
When oxygen is in use, cigarette smoking is not allowed and 'Hazard' notices are prominently displayed in the patient's room. If spanners (wrenches) are needed for oxygen tanks, 'non-sparking' wrenches must be used. Heating pads and other electrical appliances are not used.

2. *Equipment*:
All equipment must be carefully put away after use so that it does not present a hazard to patients who are ambulatory.
It is essential that a clear pathway is maintained between the patient's bed and the toilet.

3. *Miscellaneous*:
Floors are kept clean and dry. If patients are confused or sedated, bed-side rails are kept in the upright position when the patient is in bed and the bed is kept in the low position. The 'nurse-call system' is always kept within easy reach of the patient.

Evaluation: Effective planned care will reduce potential safety hazards and prevent the patient from acquiring nosocomial infections.

8. The need for personal cleansing and dressing

Potential problems	Origin of problem
8.1 poor oral hygiene	dehydration
	infection
	lethargy
8.2 inadequate body hygiene	confusion
	incontinence
	immobility

Objectives of care
1. To maintain good oral hygiene

2.   To preserve the integrity and cleanliness of the integumentary system

Nursing intervention

Mouth care: Ambulatory patients should be encouraged to brush their teeth with a soft toothbrush after each meal and taught how to use dental floss or dental tape to keep the teeth clean. Glycerine and lemon swabs may be used. Mouthwash solution is useful for patients who have a dry mouth or halitosis. Candidiasis ('thrush') is a common opportunist infection in patients with AIDS/ARC, requiring treatment with antifungal preparations, such as topical applications of nystatin oral suspension or amphotericin lozenges. In patients with AIDS/ARC, systemic anti-fungal medication may be needed. Drugs used for this include **amphotericin**, orally or by intravenous infusion, and **ketoconazole**, orally. *Candida oesophagitis* may occur as well as disseminated candidiasis in some patients with AIDS.

Body hygiene: The patient should have a daily bath or shower. If confined to bed, a daily bed-bath is required. Patients who are ambulatory, should be encouraged to dress in clean outdoor clothes for part of the day. Patients who have fever and/or night sweats, may need assistance in washing after an episode of sweating, requiring careful drying and a change of night clothes and bed linen. Talcum powder after washing is often soothing.

Pressure area care: Two-hourly pressure area care is required for patients confined to bed, as described above.

Infection control: Patients who have skin lesions and cannot use the shower, should have an antibacterial agent, such as Triclosan 2% ('Ster–Zac' bath concentrate – Hough, Hoseason & Co., Ltd.), in their bath to prevent secondary infection. Personal clothing which becomes contaminated can safely be disinfected by washing in a washing machine with ordinary detergents, on the hot cycle. Patients should have their own toothbrush and razor. These should not be shared with anyone else. An electric razor may be useful, especially if the patient has a bleeding disorder.

Evaluation: The patient remains clean and dry and the integument intact. Candidiasis is controlled.

9. The need for expression and communication

Potential problems	**Origin of problem**
9.1 impaired cognition disorientation	neurological consequences of infection with HIV or CNS opportunistic disease
9.2 isolation	fear of AIDS by family, friends, health care workers excessive IC precautions

Objectives of care
1. To minimize the effects of neurological dysfunction
2. To prevent the deleterious effects of social isolation

Nursing intervention

Assessment: Establish the status of the patient's orientation to time, place and events. Document visitors the patient wishes to see (and any he does not wish to see).

Visitors: Caring for the patient's visitors is often a delicate task, especially if they do not know the patient's diagnosis or sexual orientation. No information on any aspect of the patient's condition may be given to any visitors without the patient's express consent. With the patient's permission, visitors should be encouraged. The special friend(s) or lover of a homosexual patient often assumes the role of the patient's next of kin, which must be respected. As always, all visitors to the hospital must be treated with respect and consistent courtesy. An officious or abrupt manner displayed by health care workers to visitors can do immeasurable damage to their willingness to visit the patient and is demoralizing to the patient. It is also an unpardonable professional transgression. If possible, visitors should be allowed throughout the day. Some patients with AIDS will have been abandoned by both friends and family. With the patient's permission, it is possible to contact voluntary support groups (e.g. The Terrence Higgins Trust) who can arrange for members from their organisation to visit the patient. The hospital's voluntary services may also be able to provide this service.

Communication aids: The patient should have easy access to a telephone, stamps and stationery. If in a single room, it may be possible for the patient to have a television set. The patient should have a bedside radio (with earphones), newspapers and magazines. The 'nurse call system' must always be within easy reach of the patient. There should be a clock and a calendar in the patient's room.

Time for talking/listening/touching: Nursing care plans must take into account the fact that patients need to talk to their nurses. Listening, holding a patient's hand and just quietly being with the patient is a necessary aspect of nursing art.

Infection control: Appropriate IC precautions, as described previously, are necessary for patients who are immunocompromised or infectious. However, excessive IC precautions represent another barrier between the patient and other human beings and must be avoided. When appropriate, the patient should be encouraged to enjoy full ward privileges and to mix with other patients.

Reality orientation: Patients who are confused must be gently reminded of their environment, day and date and reassured that they are safe. They must not be spoken to as if they were children. It is generally useful if first names are used when speaking to the patient unless he has objected to this. There is nothing wrong in nurses using their own first names when talking to patients. Patients often relate better to health care workers when allowed to use their first names rather than using 'Nurse Adams' or 'Miss Williamson.'

Evaluation: A plan of care which is designed to allow patients both space and time to communicate with their families, friends and health care workers will reduce the sense of loneliness, rejection and isolation felt by many patients with AIDS.

10.   The need for working and playing

Potential problems   **Origin of problem**
10.1   Economic hardship   loss of employment
10.2   Mental deterioration   boredom, CNS involvement,
                                       loneliness

Objectives of care
1.   To provide access to appropriate financial resources
2.   To minimize effects of boredom and loneliness

Nursing intervention

Assessment: Effects of absence from usual employment are assessed and the nursing history documents the patient's neurological status and the presence of any sensory deficits or physical disablement. The history should include information relating to the patient's past leisure time activities, hobbies and interests. It is important to assess if the patient expects visits from family and significant others (lover, friends) or if he has been abandoned.

Financial problems: It is probable that all patients with long term illness, including AIDS, will eventually need to claim various State benefits to which they are entitled. As the Social Security System is confusing and complex, the patient should be interviewed by a social worker as soon as possible. Table 7.2 indicates some of the benefits to which patients may be entitled.

Table 7.2 Benefits

UK	USA
Supplementary Benefit	Supplemental Social Security Insurance (SSI)
Unemployment Benefit	
Statutory Sick Pay	Social Security Disability Insurance (SSDI)
Sickness Benefit	
Invalidity Pension & allowance	Various City & State Benefits
Housing Benefits	Veteran's Benefits
Private Insurance	Private Insurance
	Medicaid
	Union benefits
	Food Stamps

In the UK, individuals with AIDS can obtain information on entitlement from the Department of Health and Social Security (DHSS) by telephoning the operator and asking for 'DHSS Freephone' or telephoning the DHSS in London on 01-407 5522. The prompt issue of medical and sickness certificates, while the patient is in hospital, is important and should not be left until the patient asks for them. The social worker may also be able to assist patients who have been dismissed by their employers as a result of illness.

Leisure time activities: It is important that patients have access to television viewing and a radio. The library services of the hospital should be introduced and arrangements made for the patient to purchase newspapers and magazines. An occupational therapy assessment may be indicated for some patients. Special interests and hobbies should be encouraged.

Visitors: Visiting times must be flexible and visitors encouraged. If the patient has no visitors, with his permission, the Volunteer Services or a voluntary organisation may be able to arrange visitors for the patient. The largest voluntary organisation in the United Kingdom for patients with AIDS is the Terrence Higgins Trust and they can be contacted by telephone on (London) 01 833 2971 (7.00–10.00 p.m. weekdays and 3.00–10.00 p.m. at weekends). It is also important for the patient to have visits from health care workers, espcially if they are being nursed in single rooms. Time must be made available to visit and talk to the patient rather than entering the room to 'do' something.

Evaluation: The patient receives all necessary assistance to deal with claiming benefit entitlements, planning leisure time activities and arranging for visitors.

11. The need for adequate rest and sleep

Potential problem
11.1   insomnia

Origin of problem
pain, discomfort or anxiety

Objective of care
1.   To ensure that the patient has uninterrupted periods of sleep

Nursing intervention

Assessment: The patient's usual sleeping environment (e.g. own or shared bed) and habits are ascertained. This includes noting the time the patient usually goes to bed, periods of wakefulness during the night and usual time of rising. Any current complaints of pain or signs of anxiety are noted.

Comfort: Noise is a frequent cause of complaint from all patients in hospital. Every effort must be made to eliminate unnecessary noise, especially during the night. This specifically includes loud talking or laughter at the nurse's station. Drinks containing caffeine (tea, coffee, colas) should be avoided after the evening meal and a hot milk drink ('Horlicks') may be useful in helping to settle the patient. If the physician allows, an alcoholic drink may be beneficial. The patient should be assisted to void before retiring and the bedlinen should be straightened. Pressure area care and a back rub are also useful in helping the patient relax before retiring. With seriously ill patients, requiring intensive nursing during the night, care should be planned so that all required care is given at one time, allowing the patient two hour periods of uninterrupted sleep. Most patients in hospital benefit from an after-noon 'rest period' shortly after lunch. Visitors should be asked not to visit during this time.

Medication: Analgesics or night sedation may be prescribed by the medical staff. Night sedation is ineffective if pain is present. Often appropriate analgesia is sufficient to allow the patient to fall asleep. The benzodiazepine group of drugs are the most useful type of hypnotics used and include nitrazepam and flurazepam. Chloral hydrate capsules, methyprylone and chlormethiazole edisylate are sometimes useful if benzodiazepines prove ineffective. Barbiturates should be avoided. Anxiety may have to be treated with anxiolytic medication such as diazepam, chlordiazepoxide or lorazepam. Early morning wakening may be a sign of clinical depression, which requires specific treatment with anti-depressant medications, such as amitriptyline Hcl, doxepin Hcl or trimipramine maleate.

Evaluation: With well planned nursing care, patients should obtain adequate rest and sleep while in hospital.

12. The need to maintain psychological equilibrium

Actual problem	Origin of problem
12.1 anxiety	stress associated with progressive, terminal illness, fear of loss of confidentiality

Potential problems	
12.2 Ineffective coping	loss of control
12.3 Social isolation	withdrawal of social supports isolation in hospital
12.4 Loss of self-esteem	guilt, altered body image, stigma of AIDS, perception of self as contagious to others
12.5 Depression	helplessness, grief associated with loss of – personal relationships – self-esteem – physical potency – control – sexuality – effective role in life

Objectives of care
1. To allow patient to ventilate feelings and emotions
2. To alleviate predisposing factors to psychological dysfunction
3. To offer support
4. To facilitate referrals to appropriate support personnel/agencies

Nursing intervention

Assessment: During the first few days of admission, the level of anxiety present can be ascertained. Loss of adequate coping mechanisms and signs or symptoms of clinical depression must be noted. The patient's general affect may change from day to day (or from shift to shift). This must be assessed and documented in order to plan effective nursing intervention.

Anxiety: Anxiety is neither inappropriate nor uncommon in a life-threatening illness such as AIDS. Manifestations of anxiety occur on several levels, ranging from mild tension to sympathetic nervous system overflow and panic. Most patients will require assistance in handling excessive anxiety.

Level 1 (Mild): The patient is alert, enquiring, relatively relaxed and defense mechanisms are working well. In this level, patients are receptive to information.

Level 2 (Moderate): Increased alertness and heightened emotional state. The patient is more receptive to sensory information than factual information and is able to learn relaxation techniques. In this level, patients are able to solve most problems on their own.

Level 3 (Severe): Sympathetic nervous system overflow is present with typical fight or flight responses. With severe anxiety, patients are no longer able to solve problems on their own, needing the advocate skills of the nurse. Physical signs and symptoms of anxiety are often present such as tachycardia, restlessness, irritability and a feeling of 'butterflies in the stomach.' He is frightened.

Level 4 (Panic): The patient is overwhelmed by fear. He is unable to concentrate, having more pronounced physical signs of sympathetic overactivity, such as insominia, tachycardia, profuse perspiration (especially on the palms and forehead), frequency of micturition and defaecation, rapid breathing and vertigo.

Patients do not progress from level 1 through to level 4, but fluctuate from one level to another. Stressful events occurring during illness may precipitate more severe levels of anxiety. Stressors in AIDS include:

- progressive debilitation
- sensational media interest
- rejection: family, lover, friends, employer
- infection control precautions ('isolation')
- discrimination
- termination of treatment
- required rapid changes in lifestyle
- progressive changes in body image
- threatened (or actual) loss of confidentiality
- growing awareness of prognosis

Intervention designed to alleviate excessive anxiety includes discussing with patients their fears, rationally highlighting their identifiable strengths to cope with stressors, and encouraging socialization and leisure time activities. Most hospitals have clinical psychologists on their staff who can offer more skilled assistance to the patient in alleviating anxiety and teaching relaxation techniques. Severe anxiety or panic generally requires anxiolytic medication, such as benzodiazepines (discussed previously). These drugs are more useful for short-term management of acute anxiety rather than long-term use.

Depression: Clinical depression is common in AIDS, and its early recognition allows prompt treatment. Patients may despair, complain of sleep disturbances (early morning wakening, difficulty in falling asleep), lose the ability to concentrate, show a loss of interest, energy and further anorexia. Ideas of self-reproach are associated with feelings of despair, hopelessness and guilt. Delusions (false, fixed beliefs) of being punished for being homosexual are common. Loss of sexual interest and impotence is frequent. Suicidal feelings may be articulated, suicide being a significant risk. Mental retardation, as seen in depression, in patients with AIDS often acts as a brake on suicidal acts but it cannot be relied upon. In general, antidepressant medication is required for all but the mildest incidents of depression.

Although there are various types of antidepressants, the **tricyclic** group of antidepressants are the safest and most commonly prescribed. These include amitriptyline, trimipramine, clomipramine and imipramine. Another group of antidepressants, known as **monoamine oxidase inhibitors (MAOI)** such as phenelzine, mebanazine and tranylcypromine, are less often prescribed. If a patient is prescribed antidepressant medication, it is imperative that the nurse is aware to which group the drug belongs. MAOI's require specific dietary restrictions as foods rich in tyramine (cheese, Bovril, Oxo, Marmite, chianti and some types of beer) may interact with these drugs and provoke a hypertensive crisis with the risk of subarachnoid haemorrhage.

MAOI's also interact with pethidine (meperidine Hcl USP), opiates, phenothiazines and alcohol. In the two to three weeks before anti-depressants become effective, the risk of suicide remains real. Anti-depressants are generally very effective. Treatment may have to continue for several months if a relapse is to be prevented.

Patient support groups: An useful way to help patients deal with the various psychological dysfunctions which may occur in AIDS, is to form support groups for those with this diagnosis. These groups are best led by a clinical psychologist who specializes in this condition or by a psychiatric nurse specialist, who has had special training in leading these groups. Following discharge, support groups can be attended on an outpatient basis.

Individual counselling and psychotherapy: In all stages of HIV infec-tion, from seroconversion to fully expressed AIDS and eventual death, individual counselling and psychotherapy will be needed. Although all physicians caring for patients with AIDS will have good counselling and basic psychotherapy skills, the advice and assistance of clinical psychologists will be needed.

Family and significant others: It is not only the patient who requires psychological and emotional support. Family, husbands and wives, lovers and friends all display various levels of anxiety. Enormous demands are commonly made upon nursing staff and the highest degree of skill and sensitivity is required.

Central nervous system disease: HIV can directly cause CNS damage, patients exhibiting signs of a slowly progressive dementia. Gross cogni-tive changes may occur. The patient will become confused and dis-oriented. Motor (lower limb weakness) and sensory (blindness) changes may occur. Opportunistic diseases (toxoplasmosis, encephalitis secondary to various opportunistic pathogens, etc.) may also occur, causing a variety of signs and symptoms, all affecting the patient's ability to maintain psychological equilibrium. Some of these diseases are treatable; many are not.

Evaluation: Psychological dysfunction should be recognised early and nursing intervention and medical treatment implemented to alleviate and contain the mental distress which the patient is suffering. Patients will be able to learn to use effective relaxation techniques. Nursing personnel will liaise closely with other care givers.

13. The need to worship according to his own faith

Potential problem   **Origin of problem**
13.1 religious deprivation   isolation, guilt

Objective of care
1. To facilitate access between patient and chaplain or religious adviser.

Nursing intervention

Assessment: The patient's religious faith and any special religious needs should be ascertained. The patient should be asked if he would like the hospital chaplain to visit him.

Facilitating worship: Chaplains and other religious advisers must, at the patient's wish, have complete access. Often patients can be taken to the hospital chapel for religious services. It is essential that Roman Catholic patients have the opportunity of attending confession and of receiving the holy sacraments. The Sacrament of the Anointing of the Sick (i.e., Extreme Unction or Last Rites) is extremely important and this event should be entered in the patient's nursing notes. The sacrament of Holy Communion is important to members of the Church of England. At the patient's request, chaplains can make available religious literature and a Bible. The opportunity to participate in religious worship is a tremendous comfort to many patients with AIDS. Patients should not be visited by religious advisers whom they have not requested to see.

Evaluation: The patient will have opportunities to worship and be comforted by his religious beliefs.

14. The need to express sexuality

Actual problem   **Origin of problem**
14.1 need to modify sexual   infectious nature of HIV
      behaviour   infection

Potential problems
14.2 loss of libido   progressive illness
14.3 development of unsafe   guilt,
      sexual behaviour   internalized
      patterns   homophobia

14.4   grief associated with loss   changing body image, loss of
        of sexuality   sexual partner

Objectives of care
1.   To help patients adjust to changing sexual status
2.   To provide patients with information on safer sex

Nursing intervention

Assessment: Ascertain patient's attitude towards sexual expression and current problems. Determine patient's knowledge of safer sex techniques.

Patient education: Many patients have immense feelings of guilt over past sexual behaviour, which may have predisposed them to infection with HIV. Christ and Wiener[10] have described five behaviour patterns some patients adopt in response to this guilt: (1) celibacy; (2) denial or rejection of facts leading to continued high levels of sexual activity; (3) celibacy with close friends while engaging in multiple anonymous sexual contacts; (4) increased use of drugs and alcohol; (5) development of small groups of sexual contacts. Some patients with AIDS have described feelings of internalized homophobia, i.e., an internalization of society's prejudicial attitudes towards homosexuals. This may lead to a belief that homosexuality caused their disease or anger and blame directed at their sexual partner(s).

Reality orientation may reinforce factual information regarding AIDS and its transmission. Some patients need reminding that AIDS is caused by a virus, not by homosexuality, and that, although homosexuals were especially vulnerable to attack by the virus in the first years of the epidemic, *all* sexually active individuals outside of monogamous relationships are at risk. *AIDS is a human disease, not a homosexual disease*. As the vast majority of individuals infected with HIV were infected several years ago before the various 'high risk' sexual activities were identified, no one individual or groups of individuals are to blame for its current pandemic status.

In the current state of knowledge, 'high risk' sexual behaviour is well established. All persons have a responsibility to modify their sexual behaviour accordingly. This includes patients with AIDS, ARC and those who know they are seropositive for anti-HIV. It also includes all sexually active individuals outside of monogamous relationships.

Table 7.3 lists current advice for 'safer sex.'

Table 7.3 Safer sex guidelines

1. Reduce the number of different individuals with whom you have sex
2. Avoid anal intercourse (active or passive)
3. Avoid oral-anal sex
4. Avoid oral-genital sex
5. Avoid deep 'wet' kissing
6. Sex toys are safe as long as they are not shared with others
7. Mutual masturbation, body rubbing and 'dry' kissing are safe
8. Use rubber condoms (rubbers) for vaginal sex outside monogamous relationships[11]
9. Use water-based lubricants (e.g. KY Jelly) with condoms. The use of water-soluble spermicide gels containing nonoxynol-9 5% ('Delfen', Ortho-Cilag) may offer further protection as this detergent spermicide can rapidly inactivate HIV (and herpes virus) in vitro. How effective this is in vivo is not yet known[12].
10. If anal intercourse cannot be given up, use condoms and water-based lubricants, or a spermicide gel containing nonoxynol-9 5%.

NB The above guidelines are for all sexually active individuals, heterosexual and homosexual

Leaflets explicitly describing safer sex practices are available from both the Health Education Council (78 New Oxford St., London WC1A 1AH) and the Terrence Higgins Trust (BM AIDS, London WC1N 3XX). In the United States, this information is available from many organisations including: The San Francisco AIDS Foundation, 333 Valencia St., San Francisco, California 94103 and GMHC, Box 274, 132 West 24th St., New York, New York 10011. These may be ordered and stocked on wards or units where patients with AIDS may be admitted and used in patient education programmes. It may be useful to give some patients the telephone number of groups which offer 'safer sex' advice. In the UK, the Terrence Higgins Trust runs an AIDS 'Help-Line' every day from 7.00 to 10.00 p.m. on (London) 01 833 2971. In the United States, the Gay Men's Health Crisis (GMHC) have an AIDS 'Hot-Line' on (New York) [212] 807 6655. This allows individuals an opportunity independently to obtain information and advice from a source they trust and reinforces patient education efforts in hospital.

If patients are given the right information, most will make the necessary changes in their lifestyle to respond responsibly to the presence of this threat in the community. Some patients with AIDS may have significant psychological dysfunction preventing them from reacting appropriately to health education efforts. In these cases, the nurse should discuss with the attending physician the advantages of a referral to a clinical psychologist who is more skilled in assisting patients adjust to the dynamics of AIDS.

Evaluation: Adequate support and educative efforts will enable the patient to adjust to his changing sexuality and modify future sexual behaviour to protect himself and others.

15. Needs associated with dying

Actual problems	**Origin of problem**
15.1 fear, anxiety and loneliness	impending death, manner of death, loss of power and control

Potential problems	
15.2 physical problems associated with dying from AIDS	pathophysiology of HIV disease
15.3 inability to adjust to impending death	fear

Objectives of care
1. To alleviate or control physical problems associated with dying from AIDS
2. To support and reassure the patient through the various psychological stages associated with death.

Nursing intervention

Assessment: Physical problems associated with AIDS affect the dying patient and include:

- pain
- dyspnoea
- nausea/vomiting
- immobility
- open lesions/wounds
- fever

- incontinence
- cough
- pressure sores
- dysphagia
- confusion
- dehydration

In assessing the dying patient, the presence of the above should be noted and care planned accordingly, as discussed previously in this chapter. It is important to ascertain the extent of the patient's knowledge about his own impending death. It is rare that a patient, seriously ill with AIDS, is unaware that he is dying. If his assessment indicates that he is, this fact should be made known to his physician, who has the primary responsibility of discussing the patient's prognosis with him. If (or when) his level of anxiety permits, practical aspects of the patient's death may be gently discussed with him. This may include referral to a legal adviser for patients who have not made a Will. It is extremely important that the nursing notes indicate who is to be informed when the patient dies. This information should come from the patient. It would be tragic simply to inform the family, when the most significant relationship may be the patient's lover.

Wills: Patients should be encouraged to make a final and legal Will. Patients requiring assistance with this should be directed to the administrative department of the hospital or to the social worker. Under *no* circumstances should nurses help draw up Wills or witness them.

Psychological stages of dying: Although it is true that no two individuals react in the same way to impending death, there seem to be commonalities in their reactions. Dr. Elisabeth Kubler-Ross has elegantly described these[13] and Table 7.4 outlines this process.

Table 7.4   The five 'Stages of Dying'

---

1.   Denial: 'No, not me.' This is a typical reaction when a patient learns that he or she is terminally ill. Denial is important and necessary. It helps cushion the impact of the patient's awareness that death is inevitable.

2.   Rage and Anger: 'Why me?' The patient resents the fact that others will remain healthy and alive while he or she must die. God is a special target for anger since He is regarded as imposing, arbitrarily, the death sentence. To those who are shocked at her claim that such anger is not only permissible but inevitable, Doctor Ross replies succinctly, 'God can take it.'

3.   Bargaining: 'Yes me, but . . .' Patients accept the fact of death but strike bargains for more time. Mostly they bargain with God – 'even among people who never talked with God before.' Sometimes they bargain with the physician.

Table 7.4   *Cont'd*

They promise to be good or to do something in exchange for another week or month or year of life. Notes Dr. Ross: 'What they promise is totally irrelevant, because they don't keep their promises anyway.'

4.   Depression: 'Yes me.' First, the person mourns past losses, things not done, wrongs committed. Then he or she enters a state of 'preparatory grief,' getting ready for the arrival of death. The patient grows quiet, does not want visitors. 'When a dying patient doesn't want to see you any more,' says Doctor Ross, 'this is a sign he has finished his unfinished business with you and it is a blessing. He can now let go peacefully.'

5.   Acceptance: 'My time is very close now and it's all right.' Dr. Ross describes this final stage as 'not a happy stage, but neither is it unhappy. It's devoid of feelings but it's not resignation, it's really a victory.'

In reality, patients go back and forth, from one stage to another, not necessarily in consecutive order. However, this model provides a good guide for the nurse in trying to understand the different phases of coming to terms with a terminal illness. In Stage 4, nurses can be helpful in reminding patients of the achievements of their lives, the impact that all human beings have by living a life however short. If the patient has not been abandoned, loved ones have time to express their love and respect, reassuring the patient that he will be remembered.

Last offices: Usual last offices are carried out. The patient is washed and the room tidied. Loved ones are allowed to see the body before further procedures are carried out. The nurse must be accessible during this time as often their grief is close to unbearable. After the body has been viewed, it is placed in a shroud and then gently placed in a heavy duty plastic body bag. Nurses must wear disposable gloves and a plastic apron when carrying out last offices. Once the body has been placed in the body bag, no further IC precautions are required.

Summary

The individualized care of patients with AIDS and HIV-related illnesses requires skill, competence and confidence. These are based on a factual understanding of the pathophysiology of HIV-infection and a comprehensive knowledge of modern models of nursing care, designed to offer all clients, regardless of race, age, creed, sex, sexual orientation or disease, the highest quality of compassionate, non-judgemental nursing care. Anything less is disreputable to the profession and discreditable to the nurse.

References

1. Henderson, V. (1964). The nature of nursing. *American Journal of Nursing* 64(8):62–68
2. Roper, N., Logan, W.W., Tierney, A.J. (1980). *The Elements of Nursing*. Churchill-Livingstone. (London)
3. Orem, D.E. (1980). *Nursing: Concepts of Practice*. 2nd ed. McGraw–Hill Book Co. (New York)
4. Henderson, V. (1964). *Basic Principles of Nursing Care*. International Council of Nurses, Geneva
5. *Ibid*.
6. Roper (1980) *op. cit*. p 17–22
7. Norton, D., McLaren, R., Exton–Smith, A. (1975). *An Investigation of Geriatric Nursing Problems in Hospital*. Churchill Livingstone, Edinburgh
8. *Ibid*.
9. Roper (1980). *op. cit*. p. 184–5
10. Christ, G.H. and Wiener, L.S. (1985). Psychosocial issues in AIDS, *in AIDS: Etiology, Diagnosis, Treatment and Prevention* ed. by DeVita, V.T. Jr., Hellman, S. and Rosenberg, S.A., J.P. Lippincott Co. (New York) p 283
11. Conant, M., Hardy, D., Sernatinger, J., Spicer, D. and Levy, J.A. (1986). Condoms prevent transmission of AIDS – associated retrovirus. *Journal of the American Medical Association* (April 4) 255(13):1706
12. Hicks, D.R., Martin, L.S., Getchell, J.P., *et al*. (1985) Inactivation of HTLV-III/LAV-infected cultures of normal human lymphocytes by Nonoxynol-9 in vitro. *Lancet* (December 21/28) ii:1422–3 and Letter – Corrections: Voeller, B. (1986) Nonoxynol-9 and HTLV-III, *Lancet* (May 17) i:1153
13. Kubler–Ross, E. (1969). *On death and dying*. Macmillan (New York)

8

Nursing in Special Departments and in the Community

Patients with HIV-related illness frequently will be cared for and treated in most departments of the hospital and in the community.

The care of patients in the operating department

The following points apply to patients in the operating department:

1. The patient should be scheduled for the end of the list, which allows time for adequate cleaning of the operating room after surgery.

2. If possible, the patient should be anaesthetized in the operating room, rather than in the anaesthetic room. All non-essential equipment should be removed from the anaesthetic machine and ventilators, if used, are fitted with a detachable autoclavable circuit and filters.

3. Careful planning is required to ensure that all equipment needed for surgery on a patient with 'blood and body fluid precautions' is available. This includes adequate supplies of:

    -   appropriate disinfectant (e.g. freshly prepared glutaraldehyde 2%)
    -   plastic aprons (which need to be worn under gowns)
    -   eye protection devices
    -   labels for specimens ('Risk of Infection' or 'BioHazard' labels)
    -   red plastic and red nylon linen bags
    -   heavy duty, yellow plastic bags

4. Non-essential personnel should not be admitted to the operating room during surgery and an extra circulating nurse should be stationed outside the door to the operating room to obtain any needed equipment or supplies during surgery. This will decrease the risk of any possible contamination from the operating room into the rest of the operating department.

5.   Circulating nurses in the operating room must wear full protective clothing. This includes gloves (non-sterile), plastic apron, gown, and eye protection.

6.   If available, disposable linen should be used for the operating table and trolley. The operating table should be covered with a waterproof sheet, which in turn is covered by a disposable sheet.

7.   The patient should be recovered in the operating room if possible.

8.   Used instruments are autoclaved before washing. After being allowed to cool, they are washed in soapy water, rinsed and re-autoclaved. Brushes used for cleaning instruments must be autoclaved or discarded.

9.   Any spillages of blood or other body fluids should be dealt with as previously described.

10.   Non-autoclavable instruments should be immersed in glutaraldehyde 2% for one hour. This solution should then be discarded and the instruments physically cleaned in warm water and detergent, rinsed and then re-immersed in glutaraldehyde 2% and left to soak for three hours.

11.   Suction bottles should contain 30 ml of glutaraldehyde 2% or 60 ml of a strong solution of hypochlorite (containing 10 000 ppm of available chlorine). After surgery, they should be carefully emptied, rinsed and autoclaved.

12.   Closed circuits from anaesthetic machines or ventilators should be removed and sent to the Central Sterile Supplies Department (CSSD) for decontamination.

13.   Only disposable anaesthetic equipment (e.g., airway pieces, masks, corrugated tubing) should be used. If these are not available, only sterilizable equipment must be used.

14.   After surgery, the operating room and all equipment must be thoroughly cleaned with hot, soapy water.

15.   It is not necessary to allocate a special operating room for patients with HIV infection.

The care of patients in the out-patients department

Patients with HIV-related illnesses may of course use the reception and waiting room facilities used by all other patients. They do *not* require segregation from patients without HIV-related disease. Venesectionists must wear a plastic apron and a pair of disposable, latex gloves when obtaining blood specimens. Nursing personnel must be informed if a patient has been diagnosed as having an HIV-related illness or is sero-positive for anti-HIV. Endoscopic procedures (sigmoidoscopies, bron-choscopies, etc.) and biopsies should be scheduled for the end of the clinic list. Usual IC precautions are taken when assisting in invasive procedures as described previously. This includes wearing an effective, high filtration mask, eye protection, a gown over a plastic apron and disposable, latex gloves. If a special room has not been set aside for dealing with HIV-related disorders, all non-essential equipment is removed from the room prior to the procedure. Suction bottles should contain 30 ml of either glutaraldehyde 2% or a strong solution of hypochlorite.

The care of the patient in the STD clinic

Many individuals infected with HIV will be initially seen in STD (sexually transmitted diseases) Clinics, which have considerable exper-tise in dealing with these patients. Because of the epidemic proportions of this infection, sensible IC precautions must be used when dealing with *all* patients seen regardless of their known serological status. This means wearing a plastic apron and a pair of disposable, latex gloves when taking blood from *any* patient in the clinic as well as the adoption of IC precautions appropriate for dealing with sharps, specimens, equipment and all invasive procedures. STD Clinics should be well stocked with explicit health education literature. This can be obtained from the Terrence Higgins Trust in the UK and from either the San Francisco AIDS Foundation or the Gay Men's Health Crisis in the USA. Health advisers play an essential role in supporting these patients. They must have the necessary training and knowledge base in order to do so. There should be a close liaison between the STD Clinic and the Department of Psychology as many individuals require extra-ordinary counselling and support.

The nursing care of patients in the community

Almost all patients with AIDS will require community nursing services at some point in their illness. It is essential that community nurses caring for patients with AIDS are free of any infectious illness (e.g.

colds, herpes labialis, etc.) so as not to transmit any infections to the client. Good handwashing technique, prior to nursing the patient and on completion of nursing care, is required. The following points should be considered when assessing and planning care for clients in the community:

1.   Community nurse managers should ensure that all equipment needed for the usual IC precautions is readily available to community nurses. This will include supplies of:

- appropriate disinfectants (a strong solution of hypochlorite solution or glutaraldehyde 2%). The usual disinfectant used by community nursing personnel is a strong hypochlorite solution (household bleach diluted one part bleach: ten parts water).
- plastic aprons
- effective, high filtration masks
- red plastic bags for contaminated linen and red, nylon bags
- sharps container
- disposable, latex gloves
- eye protection devices
- heavy duty, yellow plastic bags
- specimen labels (i.e., 'Risk of Infection' or 'BioHazard' labels)

2.   Any cuts or open lesions on the arms or hands of nursing personnel must be covered with a waterproof, occlusive plaster (tape). Nurses with eczema should not deliver care to patients with HIV-related illnesses.

3.   No protective clothing or IC precautions are required to enter the patient's home, for introductions (shaking his hand) and talking to the patient.

4.   A home-care nursing assessment should be carried out prior to the patient's discharge from hospital. The community nurse should visit the patient while he is still in hospital, assist in advising on discharge planning and discuss the care requisites with the patient's general practitioner as soon as the referral is received.

5.   The actual delivery of nursing care to this client is exactly the same as for any other client, with the added adoption of sensible and appropriate IC precautions, *when necessary*. Additional services may be required such as home helps, 'meals-on-wheels' and other relevant social services. The community nurse should be aware of the range of services available from voluntary organisations, such as the Terrence

Higgins Trust and discuss the possible advantages of these with the patient.

6. Used linen contaminated with blood or body secretions can be washed by the patient, his family or friends in a standard washing machine on a hot cycle. If the patient lives alone and is too ill to do this, contaminated linen may be sent to the local authority laundry service, double-bagged in red water soluble plastic bags ('alginate' stitched or polyvinyl alcohol) inside red, nylon bags. Used linen which is not contaminated with blood or body fluids may be washed in the usual way.

7. Contaminated rubbish is placed inside heavy duty, yellow plastic bags, carefully sealed and sent for incineration. A waterproof, puncture-resistant plastic sharps container must be kept in the patient's home. When it is three-quarters full, it is sealed and placed in a heavy duty, yellow plastic bag and sent for incineration. Different health authorities have varied procedures for sending material for incineration. The community nurse must be familiar with the procedure for his/her own authority. Usually, arrangements are made for collection through the local environmental health department. It is important that red bags of contaminated linen and sealed yellow bags of infected rubbish are *not* left outside the patient's door for collection. Neighbours quickly become curious, which may be an added stress for the client. They should be left just inside the front door and the collection services instructed to ring the door-bell or knock on the door. Collection service personnel do *not* need to wear any protective clothing as linen or infectious material sealed in the appropriate bag represents no further IC risk.

8. The patient should be instructed not to share his tooth brush or razor with other members of the household. He does *not* require separate crockery or cutlery unless he has an oral or enteric infection. The patient can use the same bathroom and washing facilities as other members of the household. It is not necessary to pour disinfectants into the toilet. If the patient has restricted mobility and cannot use the toilet, a bedside commode or 'chemical' toilet may be useful. Bedpans and urinals are carefully emptied into the toilet (avoiding splashing), rinsed and stored dry. Soaking in disinfectants is not required. Any spillages are dealt with as previously described.

9. Community nursing personnel must wear disposable latex gloves and a plastic apron when delivering direct patient care. The need for additional protective clothing is extremely rare in a home-care setting,

although it may be required with terminally ill patients, who wish to remain at home during the final stages of their illness.

10.   The patient should be encouraged to remain as independent as possible. He can use the public library, local pub, restaurants, hairdressers and other public places, like any other member of the community. Patient education regarding 'safer sex' requires reinforcing. The patient should be advised to be discreet regarding his diagnosis. Although, in the past, patients have been advised to inform their dental practitioner of their antibody status, this is probably irrelevant. Dentists have now been instructed to adopt standard IC precautions for *all* patients, regardless of their known antibody status. Further, there have been unfortunate incidents when patients have, as advised, informed their dentist of their diagnosis and, subsequently, have been refused care.

11.   The patient should be encouraged to maintain social relationships and not to become isolated. Family and friends frequently require reassurance regarding the infectious nature of the patient's illness.

12.   If death occurs at home, the patient's general practitioner must notify the undertaker of infection hazards. Usual last offices are carried out, the patient being placed in a shroud and then in a plastic cadaver bag. The family should be advised to view the body prior to its removal by the undertakers. Embalming is not carried out for individuals who have died and are known to have been anti-HIV seropositive.

The care of the patient in the obstetric service

In assessing and planning for antenatal care, labour and delivery and the post-partum care of women who are anti-HIV seropositive, the following points should be considered:

1.   Pregnancy in an asymptomatic, anti-HIV seropositive woman is a known co-factor to the development of fully expressed AIDS. There is also a high probability of infection *in utero* to the child. The child may also become infected at the time of delivery. If this occurs, it is likely that the child will develop fully expressed AIDS as his/her immune system is not fully developed. Women in the currently known 'at risk' groups for HIV infection, may request serological screening for anti-HIV and, if positive, may be offered a termination of pregnancy.

2.   In women known to be seropositive for anti-HIV, pre-delivery (intrapartum) care is best delivered in a single room, due to the potential risks of bleeding and membrane rupture.

3.   IC precautions, as previously described for invasive procedures, are implemented during labour and delivery. This includes the wearing of plastic aprons under gowns, effective high filtration masks and eye protection.

4.   Fetal blood samples, intrauterine catheters and fetal scalp electrodes should be avoided in order to reduce the risk of transmitting HIV infection to the child.

5.   After examination, the placenta should be placed in a heavy duty, yellow plastic bag, which is sealed and sent for incineration. All specimens, including cord blood, must be labelled with the appropriate hazard labels ('Risk of Infection' or 'BioHazard' labels); the specimen request form must be similarly labelled and specimens placed in a double plastic bag, the request form being kept separate from the specimen.

6.   It is good practice to list in the patient's records all medical and nursing personnel involved in the delivery.

7.   In the postnatal period, mucus extractors must not be used on the infant. Any neonatal contact with blood or body fluids (e.g. cord stump care, heel pricks, etc.) require the usual IC precautions for patients with 'Blood and Body Fluid Precautions'. In caring for the mother, nursing personnel must adopt the previously described general IC precautions when exposure to blood or body fluids is anticipated. This includes perineal care and exposure to lochia and breast milk.

8.   As HIV has been isolated in breast milk, breast feeding is contraindicated.

9.   Disposable napkins should be used and disposed of in heavy duty, yellow plastic bags.

10.   Standard IC precautions for patients on 'Blood and Body Fluid Precautions' as previously described, are implemented in caring for the child and mother during the postnatal period.

Caring for patients in the accident and emergency department

The serological status of patients admitted to the accident and emergency department will be unknown to the nursing staff responsible for their care. As large numbers of individuals in the community can be expected to have been infected with HIV, IC precautions designed for HIV infected patients must be adopted for *all* patients requiring examination and treatment. In general, this includes wearing plastic aprons and disposable gloves when exposure to blood and body fluids is anticipated with *any* patient. Obviously 'mouth-to-mouth' resuscitation is never appropriate in a hospital emergency department and resuscitation equipment (airways, endotracheal tubes) should either be disposable or sterilizable, preferably by autoclaving. In emergency situations where gross exposure to blood or body fluids is likely (e.g. serious trauma, haematemesis), gowns (with a plastic apron worn underneath), gloves, masks and eye protection should be worn.

Caring for patients in the intensive care unit

The risk of exposure to blood or body fluids is increased in intensive care units and all of the IC precautions previously described must be implemented. Maximum use should be made of disposable equipment. Non-disposable equipment must be sterilizable. It can no longer be assumed that any blood or body fluid from any patient is 'safe,' i.e. HIV-free, and reasonable IC precautions should be incorporated into the planned care of *all* patients. Vascular access sites on *all* patients should be covered with a waterproof dressing. Diligent care must be taken with *all* sharps. The manufacturer's instructions should be followed in sterilizing ventilation equipment.

Summary

There are two important issues to consider in assessing, planning and implementing the nursing care of patients with HIV-related illnesses in the various special departments of the hospital.

1.   All departments can safely and competently care for any patient suffering from an infectious disease (including HIV infection) by adopting the general IC precautions outlined previously. In some departments, they will require modification and elaboration, depending on the level of anticipated risk of exposure to blood and body fluids.

2.   It should now be clear that it is no longer appropriate to assume that blood or body fluids from any patient are risk-free. Regardless of the known HIV serological status of the patient, routine IC precautions must be implemented for *all* patients, aimed at preventing nursing personnel coming into direct contact with blood or body fluids.

References

DHSS (1986). Guidance for surgeons, anaesthetists, dentists and their teams in dealing with patients infected with HTLV-III. *CMO(86)7 (April) Acquired Immune Deficiency Syndrome – AIDS. Booklet 3.* London

RCN Working Party (1985). *Nursing Guidelines on the management of patients in hospital and the community suffering from AIDS.* Royal College of Nursing, London (updated 1986)

9

Issues and the Management of Strategic Nursing Care

The efficient delivery of individualized patient care requires informed, insightful nursing management. The failure to develop competent and compassionate management services results in a breakdown of direct patient care, confusion and low morale among nursing staff, distress and isolation for the patient and a negative image of the hospital. Most metropolitan hospitals now have some experience in caring for patients suffering from HIV-related disease. In the beginning of the epidemic, a general commonality in problems and issues emerged. A core of expertise has now developed which other hospitals can use to avoid the early problems associated with the admission of a patient with AIDS[1].

Co-ordination of nursing care

Nursing management should initiate the formation of an 'AIDS Co-ordinating Committee,' which should have broad educational and supportive responsibilities. The committee should be composed of both experts and non-experts and be representative of the hospital community. A typical Co-ordinating Committee might have the following membership:

Experts
Infection Control Nurse
Microbiologist
Clinical Nurse Specialist
    [Medical/Oncology Nursing]
Dietitian
Physician
Clinical Psychologist
Clinical Nurse Specialist
    [Psychiatric Nursing]
Nursing In-service Instructors
Social worker/Health Adviser
Community Nurse

Non-Experts
Key Trade Union Representatives
Hospital Chaplain
Representative from Domestic/
    Housekeeping services
Representative from Transport/
    Portering Services
Senior Nurse – Occupational
    Health Services
Unit General Manager or deputy
Senior Nurse Manager

The committee must have visible and aggressive support from both nursing and hospital management and from experts within the hospital. The co-ordinating committee should have three major areas of responsibilities:

(1)   The formation and adoption of sane IC procedures as well as the monitoring of their implementation

(2)   Planning and implementing in-service education and training programmes for all grades of staff

(3)   Advising general management on policy and long-term planning for patients with HIV-related illnesses

Hospitals which currently have little experience in caring for patients with HIV-related illnesses, should form a co-ordinating committee and initiate planning prior to admitting their first patient. It is inconceivable that any general hospital will not be responsible for caring for these patients in the future. Planning now will dissipate initial anxiety and confusion.

In-service education

Hospitals which have developed aggressive in-service educational programmes for their staff have been the most successful in minimizing anxiety and disruption when a patient with HIV disease is admitted. In-service education should commence with orientation/induction of new staff and be on-going. A combination of various formats is the most useful approach, including workshops, seminars, study days and ward-based discussions and tutorials. In-service instructors and the infection control nurse are ideally placed to implement educational programmes, advised by the AIDS co-ordinating committee. A study day once a year on 'AIDS' is not adequate to deal with the new problems and issues posed by the admission of patients with HIV disease.

Infection control nurse

If not already in post, the recruitment of a clinical nurse specialist in infection control is absolutely essential. Comprehensive, competent and safe patient care, both in hospital and at home, cannot be ensured without the support and advice of this specialist. With the advent of HIV disease, it would seem impossible to cope without the guidance of an IC nurse.

Conditions of employment

Contracts of employment for all health care workers must clearly preclude the withdrawal of care from any patient, regardless of age, sex, sexual orientation, race, religion or presenting illness. Nursing management must make it absolutely clear that nursing personnel do not have the right to choose whom they will or will not nurse. Management must be seen to be determined to enforce this correct obligation of employment. Staff who are reluctant to care for a patient, should be counselled and given additional in-service training. If their reluctance persists, they should be dismissed. Quality assurance strategies should be designed to ensure that patients are not suffering as a result of ignorance, prejudice or unethical and judgemental attitudes projected onto them by health care workers.

Dedicated wards and clinics

Metropolitan hospitals experiencing significant admissions of patients with HIV-related disease should consider the creation of dedicated units. The advantages of these units include:

(1) Nursing care can be 'state of the art' and specialized care strategies can be developed to meet the complex psycho-social-medical issues seen in these patients.

(2) Most patients with HIV-related illness prefer being cared for in a dedicated unit.

(3) Motivated, concerned staff, comfortable with their own sexuality, can be recruited to these units and given additional specialist training. They will quickly gain knowledge of other available resources to enable them to formulate effective, early discharge planning.

(4) Units are cost-effective and have a positive impact on bed availability. Effective discharge planning, centralized care and the identification of other resource issues can most efficiently take place within these units.

(5) Units can attract additional funds from concerned groups in the community. There can be a positive public relations impact in their creation.

(6) The body of knowledge upon which the profession is based can be increased by the expanding expertise acquired by the nursing staff in these units.

(7) Personnel problems are minimized and hospitals which have created these units have experienced high staff morale and a correspondingly high level of patient satisfaction.

Dedicated units must have clear admission criteria and therapeutic objectives. Their existence does not mean that patients with AIDS will not be cared for in other areas of the hospital. Many patients with HIV-related illness do not require the intensive specialist care offered by dedicated units. Hospice and terminal care facilities should also be considered as dedicated units are generally designed as active treatment units. A dedicated unit will not be effective unless it is supported by a comprehensive dedicated out-patients clinic. These clinics should be able to screen patients, initiate diagnostic procedures and maintain out-patients by providing a range of services which include intravenous rehydration, blood transfusions and intravenous chemotherapy. Clinical nurse specialists need to be recruited and trained for dedicated clinics.

Counselling services and support groups

Hospitals need to develop comprehensive counselling services for patients with HIV-related disease. Although a multi-disciplinary approach is needed for the complex problems seen in this disease, clinical psychologists have the most relevant skills and should lead the planning and implementation of these services. Health advisers, social workers and lay counsellors from concerned community groups (e.g. The Terrence Higgins Trust, London) can complement this service. If lay counsellors are used, facilities must be made available to them. Counselling is required at all stages of illness, from pre-screening counselling to bereavement support, both for in-patients and for out-patients. If a hospital is treating more than a few patients with HIV-related illnesses, a patient's 'Support Group' can be established. These groups are invaluable in providing space for ventilating emotions and offering mutual support. They can include both in-patients and out-patients. Hospitals which have large numbers of patients with AIDS and other HIV-related conditions often provide a sophisticated range of support groups. For example, patients with Kaposi's sarcoma may form one group as they have specific problems coping with alterations in body image which patients with opportunistic infections may not have. Intravenous substance abusers often respond only where other group members are also substance abusers. In addition, *staff support groups* are used to provide an opportunity for health care workers to explore their anxieties, frustrations and other related 'burn-out' problems. Support groups must be competently and sensitively led by a staff member especially trained for this role.

Confidentiality

Nursing management must be sensitive to the balance required between ensuring appropriate IC precautions and the need to ensure appropriate confidentiality. The IC precautions required for safe care of all patients must be communicated to all grades of staff. This does *not* include the patient's diagnosis, which is confidential to the patient and those health care workers providing direct patient care.

Public relations

Contact with the media presents both potential problems and opportunities for the hospital to assume a leadership role in health education. In dealing with the press, precise and honest information will diminish adverse publicity. It is useful if an expert and authoritative representative of the hospital staff is designated as the spokesperson for the hospital on all HIV related issues. All hospital staff members should be required to co-ordinate all press communications through this individual. Maximum use should be made of written press releases when information is requested rather than verbal interviews, which are often 're-interpreted' by the media. The overriding principle of public relations is the maintenance of patient confidentiality and dignity.

Screening for anti-HIV

Since 1985, blood tests have been available which are capable of detecting the presence of antibodies to HIV. A positive result indicates that an individual (1) has previously been infected by HIV and (2), in the present state of knowledge, is presumed to be currently infected and infectious. It cannot predict which patients infected will progress to fully expressed AIDS. It is known that many will not. However, as the epidemic is still relatively young, it is not known if all infected individuals will eventually manifest signs of ill-health as a result of HIV infection. It is well within the realms of reality to consider that they might. A negative test for anti-HIV indicates very little. It most certainly does *not* imply that the individual is free from HIV infection. This is due to five possibilities:

(1) There can be a lag between exposure and seroconversion. Although this may be only a few weeks, it may extend up to six months. During this time, the individual will test anti-HIV negative but is infected and infectious.

(2) An individual may be free of HIV infection and test negative for anti-HIV. However, he may be exposed the following day and then become infected and infectious.

(3) Some individuals who are infected with HIV, fail to demonstrate antibodies detectable by the current serological tests and will test negative. However, they too are infected and infectious.

(4) The result may be a 'false-negative' and this patient remains infected and infectious.

(5) Some patients with fully expressed AIDS cease to produce antibodies to HIV detectable by the present generation of serological tests and eventually will test negative. However, they remain infected and infectious.

Although a positive anti-HIV test will alert nursing personnel to the need for 'Blood and Body Fluids Precautions,' a negative test is meaningless from an IC point of view. With the large and exponentially increasing numbers of individuals in the community infected with HIV, it is clear that now more than ever, 'Blood and Body Fluid Precautions' must be adopted on *all* patients. A casual approach to exposure to blood and body fluids is no longer possible in any setting, least of all a health care situation. The indications for screening for anti-HIV are limited to:

(1) All donor blood must be screened
(2) Transplant donors and donors of semen are screened
(3) Patients in haemodialysis units should be screened
(4) Rarely, screening is required for diagnostic purposes (AIDS is a clinical diagnosis, not a serological diagnosis)
(5) Women in the 'current' high risk groups should be offered screening if they are considering pregnancy
(6) Screening should be available, on demand, for individuals, who are worried that they may be infected with HIV. This is to ensure that they do not present to the Blood Transfusion Services for 'indirect' screening purposes.

True informed consent is required prior to screening. This includes explaining to the patient why screening is needed and carefully discussing the results with him. Counselling services are required for both pre- and post-screening. If these are not available, screening should not take place. Absolute confidentiality must be guaranteed as the unauthorized disclosure of this information is illegal and unethical. Information regarding test results can adversely affect a patient's relationships with his family, friends and lover, can preclude an application for life insurance resulting in a mortgage application being refused and can affect his current or future employment. In the UK, this information is *legally* confidential, protected under the terms of the National Health Service (Venereal Diseases) Regulations 1974 (SI 1974.9), and is *professionally* confidential, protected by the Code of Professional Conduct issued by the United Kingdom Central Council for Nursing, Midwifery and Health Visiting. Equally important, the unauthorized disclosure of this information is *morally* wrong. The patient's express permission must be obtained before this information is conveyed to anyone including the patient's family, general practitioner or dentist. Nursing management must ensure that mechanisms exist which can protect the patient's right to confidentiality.

There are no indications for or benefits of routine screening of health care workers. This should not be done.

Employment of health care workers who are infected with HIV

Currently, many hospitals have experienced situations where a member of their staff has developed AIDS/ARC or is asymptomatically sero-positive for anti-HIV. This has included surgeons, dentists, nurses and ancillary staff. Excluding the three or four documented incidents of gross needle-stick injuries (discussed previously), these health care workers acquired HIV infection sexually. It seems probable that, in time, all sexually active individuals may be 'at risk' for HIV infection, including health care workers. Although the occupational risk of HIV transmission is minimal (or nil if the strategies outlined in this text are diligently followed), health care workers are members of the broader community and are as much at risk sexually as any other member of the community.

As it is inconceivable that routine screening for anti-HIV could ever be implemented, most individuals who are seropositive for anti-HIV will be unknown to the employing health authority. However, occasionally this information is made known to the health authority by the employee. More commonly, health care workers who develop clinical manifestations of HIV infection consult the occupational health services and, eventually, a diagnosis of AIDS or ARC is established. Early in the epidemic, some hospitals and health authorities reacted inappropriately to this situation by suspending or dismissing the employee on the grounds that they posed an unacceptable IC risk to the patients of the hospital. This is quite clearly wrong and several issues need to be addressed in establishing the correct response of an employing health authority faced with this increasingly common predicament.

(1) The means of transmission for HIV are well established and well documented. Other than intravenous substance abuse, HIV infection is now almost exclusively a sexually transmitted disease. In a health care setting, person-to-person transmission of HIV, from a health care worker to a patient, could probably only be achieved by sexual transmission. This would be an unusual, if not a bizarre event, in hospital.

(2)   Consequently, there have been no known cases of HIV transmission from an infected health care worker to a patient.

(3)   If a health care worker was infected with HIV, it would be essential that appropriate precautions were taken to eliminate any possibility of blood or body fluid contamination from the employee to a patient. This would include covering any cuts or abrasions on the hands with a waterproof dressing and wearing disposable gloves when engaging in direct patient care. Well established, appropriate precautions should also be taken to prevent transmission of any infection (e.g. herpes) to a patient. However, all of the precautions required amount to no more than good clinical practice, which all health care workers have a responsibility to maintain, *regardless* of their serological status for anti-HIV.

(4)   Health care workers involved in invasive procedures, such as surgery, obstetrics or dentistry, may be thought to be more of a risk to patients if they are anti-HIV positive. Concern has been expressed that these health care workers should be reassigned to clinical duties, which do not involve invasive procedures. Since it will never be known with any degree of accuracy which employees are seropositive, a dilemma is immediately posed. What is the value to the patient in preventing a known seropositive health care worker carrying out invasive procedures when other health care workers may be equally seropositive but unknown to the health authority? The answer is, of course, none. Even if screening tests were 100 per cent sensitive and specific, they would have to be done on a *daily* basis to ensure that the serological status of all health care workers was known to the health authority. Even then, as previously discussed, some individuals infected with HIV will test negative for anti-HIV. Some false negatives are also likely to occur.

(5)   Another approach suggested is to screen for members of currently known 'at risk' groups, e.g. male homosexuals and intravenous substance abusers. Once identified, they could either be reassigned to duties which did not involve direct patient contact, dismissed or not employed in the first place. Other than self-disclosure, there is no way of accurately or realistically identifying either intravenous substance abusers (few of whom actually work in the health services) or homosexuals. To attempt to do so would not only be distasteful but also ethically, morally and legally unacceptable in a free society. It would be counter-productive, provoking an unprecedented witch hunt.

All strategies designed to ensure that no health care workers are infected with HIV are flawed. Further, they are unnecessary.

As we now must accept that blood and body fluids from all patients pose a potential infection risk and must take appropriate precautions, we must equally assume that blood and body fluids from all health care workers pose a potential infection risk, and must ensure that high standards of clinical practice are maintained. This is all that is necessary. There is nothing new in this approach. It has never been acceptable for health care workers to share, either directly or indirectly, their blood or body fluids with patients in their care. It is useful to keep the risk in perspective. If a nurse cuts herself or himself while delivering direct patient care, the blood from the nurse would have to gain entry to the bloodstream of the patient for a risk of infection to be realised. This is unlikely. Even in surgery or dentistry, where it could conceivably happen, the dilemma of knowing who is and who is not infected with HIV remains.

All health care workers have an individual responsibility to maintain high standards of hygiene and clinical practice. The promotion of these standards is an appropriate task of in-service education.

If a health care worker is clinically ill as a result of HIV infection, then he must be assessed on an individual basis. He is either fit for duty or is not. If he is fit for duty, then he does not need to be reassigned to other clinical areas because he is an infection risk to patients. He may require reassignment, however, to protect him from acquiring additional opportunistic infections. This decision must be made by the occupational health services and/or the employee's own personal physician. The absolute obligations of confidentiality apply equally to patients and to health care workers. Other than the employee's fitness for duty, no information is shared by the occupational health services with management. It is not only unnecessary to do so, but is wrong. If employees feel that they cannot trust the occupational health services to maintain confidentiality, they will avoid using their services.

Patient's Bill of Rights

Nursing management should construct and communicate widely a philosophy of care with which both the patient and the nurse can identify. This philosophy should include a description of the patient's rights[2]. These rights should guarantee to all patients:

(1) The right to quality health care in an atmosphere of human dignity without regard to age, ethnic or national origin, sex or sexual orientation, religion or presenting illness.
(2) The right to receive emergency medical and surgical treatment.
(3) The right to considerate, dignified and respectful care by all health care workers, regardless of the patient's physical or emotional condition.

(4) The right to be informed of the name, title and function of anyone involved in their care.

(5) The right to receive upon request an explanation of their current medical condition in language that they can understand.

(6) The right to give or decline true informed consent and to participate in the choice of treatment. If consent for treatment is not given, the right to be informed of the likely medical consequences of their action.

(7) The right to privacy to an extent consistent with providing dignified medical and nursing care.

(8) The right to confidentiality.

(9) The right to be informed and to participate in their discharge planning.

(10) The right to refuse to participate in research projects.

(11) The right to receive, upon request, a consultation and/or care and treatment from another appropriate physician on the staff other than the one assigned to them.

(12) The right, both as a patient and as a citizen, free from restraint, interference, coercion, discrimination or reprisal, to voice grievances and complaints and to recommend changes in policies and services. This implies that patients have access upon request to senior nurse managers.

(13) The right to expect visitors to be treated with courtesy and respect.

Resuscitation

In the current state of knowledge, patients with AIDS have a terminal illness. While it may be appropriate to offer ventilation and other life-support systems to patients with AIDS in the early stages, it is often not compassionate to do so in the end-stage of their illness. The patient must be involved in decisions regarding intensive care and resuscitation. It is the physician's primary responsibility to discuss this with the patient and to make the final decision. This decision must be clearly communicated to all health care workers directly involved with the care of the patient and is appropriately discussed at routine, multidisciplinary case conferences.

Summary

The competent and compassionate management of nursing is as important as the direct nursing care delivered at the bedside. The issues discussed in this chapter must not come as a surprise to management. Effective forward planning will facilitate the smooth running of the hospital and the delivery of quality care to all patients when patients with AIDS are admitted. Although each nurse is accountable for his/her own clinical and professional practice, nurse managers are individually accountable for providing adequate staffing levels, planning, guidance, formation of policies and procedures and for providing a philosophy of leadership, which promotes the high standards of care that all patients have a right to expect.

References

1. Eickhoff, T.C., *et al.* (1984). Special Report: A hospitalwide approach to AIDS - Recommendations of the Advisory Committee on Infections Within Hospitals (American Hospital Association). *Infection Control.* 5(5):242–8
2. New York City Health and Hospitals Corporation (1984). *Patient's Bill of Rights.* Office of Patient Relations, New York, USA

Further reading

1. DHSS (1985). Information for doctors concerning the introduction of the HTLV III antibody test. Acquired Immune Deficiency Syndrome – AIDS, Booklet 2 CMO(85)12, London

2. Viele, C.S., Dodd, M.J. and Morrison, C. (1984). Caring for Acquired Immune Deficiency Syndrome patients, *Oncology Nursing Forum.* (May/June) 11(3):56–60

3. Miller, D., Jeffries, D.J., Green, J., Harris, J.R.W., Pinching, A.J. (1986). HTLV-III: Should testing ever be routine? *British Medical Journal* (April 5), 292:941–943

10

The Medical Treatment of HIV Infection

With the recognition of HIV as the causative agent of AIDS and AIDS-related complex (ARC), medical research has progressed rapidly on two fronts: towards the development of an effective treatment regime and the discovery and deployment of a biological vaccine.

Medical treatment

Effective treatment would require both the destruction or inactivation of the virus in the body and the re-stimulation of the immune system.

Antiviral agents

HIV contains an enzyme, 'reverse transcriptase,' which is necessary for viral replication. Several antiviral agents are capable of inhibiting this enzyme and are being investigated for their usefulness in the treatment of HIV infections.

Suramin (suramin hexasodium salt).   This drug was developed shortly after World War I to treat African trypanosomiasis (Sleeping Sickness) and onchocerciasis (River Blindness). When given to patients with AIDS, it has been shown to inhibit the activity of reverse transcriptase with subsequent slowing of viral replication. It is usually given as one gram, intravenously, once a week. It may have to be given indefinitely for clinical improvement to be maintained[1,2]. Side effects include: nausea, vomiting, fever, oedema, headache, joint pains, ocular symptoms and cutaneous hyperesthaesia of the soles and palms. Rarely, collapse and sudden death have been associated with its use.

HPA-23 (antimoniotungstate).   This agent is a competitive inhibitor of reverse transcriptase, having anti-viral activity against a wide range of RNA and DNA viruses. It is given intravenously (e.g. 200 mg in 250 ml isotonic glucose over three hours each day for 15 days) and, like suramin, is capable of clearing the blood of detectable HIV activity. Side effects include fever and a reversible thrombocytopenia.

Foscarnet (phosphonoformate). This agent is a non-competitive inhibitor of reverse transcriptase and shows great promise. It is administered intravenously and is associated with minimal toxicity[3]. It is also useful in the treatment of cytomegalovirus infection in patients with AIDS.

Ribavirin. This agent, which is effective against many RNA viruses, is taken orally and is relatively non-toxic. It is currently being investigated for treating patients with AIDS[4].

AZT 509 (azidothymidine). Great excitement surrounds the clinical trials now under way with this new drug developed by Burroughs-Wellcome. AZT, a thymidine analogue with potent anti-viral activity against HIV, can be administered either orally or intravenously. This agent is able to cross the blood-brain barrier. It seems relatively free from serious side-effects and is not only virustatic, but also may promote partial immunological reconstitution in some patients[5]. AZT is the subject of intense medical research and public interest.

Other possibilities for intervention include monoclonal antibodies, amantadine, cellular DNA polymerase inhibitors and interferon[6].

The major difficulty currently being encountered is that, while it may be possible to clear the blood of HIV with antiviral drugs, active virus invariably returns shortly after treatment has been discontinued. Further, in patients with fully expressed AIDS, a reduction in active viral replication does not necessarily imply clinical improvement.

Immunosuppressant therapy

HIV infects some but certainly not all T4 helper cells. When these cells are stimulated, for example by antigens (STD infections) or allo-antigens (allogeneic sperm, isoantigenic material in concentrated factor VIII), infected T4 helper cells may provoke an **autoimmune disease**. Each time T4 helper cells are stimulated, there is a further autoimmune destruction of both infected and non-infected T4 cells. Immunosuppressive drugs, such as cyclosporin A, are being investigated as one means of controlling this possible autoimmune mechanism in patients with AIDS. However, immunosuppressant therapy in a patient with HIV infection is potentially dangerous and most scientific opinion is cautious regarding this approach[7].

Immune stimulation or reconstruction

As the primary defect in patients with HIV-related illness is a depressed immune system, investigators have explored the role of immuno-

stimulants such as **interleukin 2** and **interferon**. As these agents also
have some antiviral effects, they have had limited usefulness in patients
with Kaposi's sarcoma. However, as they stimulate T4 helper cells,
viral replication and disease progression is accelerated[8]. Immuno-
stimulant agents may be useful in the future, combined with effective
antiviral therapy.

Immune reconstruction, by using bone marrow grafts or leukocyte
transfusions, have not been effective as they rapidly become reinfected
with HIV.

A vaccine against HIV infection

Despite massive health education efforts, HIV infection will continue
to spread until a safe and effective vaccine is discovered. Although this
is proving to be extremely difficult, it should be possible. A vaccine has
been produced for one retrovirus, the feline leukaemia virus, which
causes a disease similar to AIDS in cats. Researchers in the United
States of America have recently been successful in inserting one of the
genes from HIV into the *Vaccinia* virus (the virus used as the basis for
the smallpox vaccine). When the altered *Vaccinia* virus is injected into
mice and rhesus monkeys, they produce antibodies against the outer
envelope of HIV, without developing AIDS[9]. This may be the first step
towards developing a vaccine for HIV infection. Approaches using
recombinant DNA, anti-idiotype antibodies and immunostimulating
complexes (iscoms) are also being explored[10, 11]. The chief difficulty in
producing a vaccine against HIV is that this retrovirus shows marked
'antigenic drift,' i.e., it keeps changing its antigenic coat. Although
medical scientists are optimistic, a vaccine may be many years away. In
the meantime, the only effective 'vaccine' is education; effective education which leads to a change in sexual behaviour designed to reduce
known risk factors associated with HIV infection.

Summary

Although impressive advances are being made in the treatment of
opportunistic diseases associated with HIV infection, scientists have
not yet developed drugs that will eliminate the virus from the body or
restore the ability of the immune system to defend the body against
repeated assaults by these pathogens. Until this has been achieved,
AIDS will continue to be a fatal disease. Immense international effort is
being directed towards the development of a vaccine against HIV but it
remains elusive.

There seems little doubt that the escape of HIV from the animal kingdom into the human population represents an uniquely sinister threat to

the human race. The advent of AIDS may turn out to be the most signif-icant event of our lifetime.

References

1. Rouvroy, D., *et al.* (1985). Short-term results with suramin for AIDS-related conditions. *Lancet.* i(April 13):878–9
2. Broder, S., Yarchoan, R., Collins, J.M., *et al.* (1985). Effects of suramin on HTLV-III/LAV infection presenting as Kaposi's Sarcoma or AIDS-Related Complex: clinical pharmacology and suppression of virus replica-tion in vivo. *Lancet.* ii(September 21):627–30
3. Sandstrom, E.G., Kaplan, J.C., Byington, R.E., Hirsch, M.S. (1985). Inhibition of human T-cell lymphotropic virus type III in Vitro by phosphonoformate, *Lancet*, i(June 29):1480–2
4. Weber, J. (1986). AIDS: the virus is not immune. *New Scientist.* January 2:37–9
5. Yarchoan, R., Klecker, R.W., Weinhold, K.J., *et al.* (1986). Administra-tion of 3'-Azido-3'-Deoxythymidine, an inhibitor of HTLV-III/LAV replication, to patients with AIDS or AIDS-related complex. *Lancet.* i(March 15):575–80
6. Weber, J. *loc. cit.*
7. Klatzmann, D. and Montagnier, L. (1986). Approaches to AIDS therapy. *Nature* 319 (January 2):10–11
8. *Ibid.*
9. Henson, N. (1986). When will we have an AIDS vaccine? *New Scientist* March 27:20
10. Francis, D.P. and Petricciani, J.C. (1985). The prospects for and path-ways toward a vaccine for AIDS. *The New England Journal of Medicine.* (December 19) 313(25):1586–90
11. Weber, J. *loc. cit.*

Index

protozoal infections 42
public relations 117
psychotherapy 96
pyrimethamine (and sulfadiazine)
47

reality orientation 90
regulator T-cells 29–30
rehydration, intravenous 79, 82
requisites for health 75–103
retrovirus 14
resuscitation 122
reverse transcriptase 14
ribavirin 125
ribonucleic acid (RNA) 12
rifampicin 46
Roper, Nancy 74–5

safer sex guidelines 99
saliva 34
salmonella typhimurium 43, 48
salmonellosis 48, 59, 63
screening 117–19
seborrheic dermatitis 42
semen 15, 17, 34
severe combined immunodeficiency
(SCID) 1, 30
sexual intercourse, anal 17
sexually transmitted diseases (STD)
15
shigella flexneri 43, 48
simian T-lymphotropic virus type-III
[STLV-III (AGM)] 17–18
skin care 82
spiramycin (Rovamycin) 47
splenomegaly 40, 42
stages of dying 101–2
state assistance and benefits 91

strategic nursing care 55, 74–5,
113–27
streptococcus pneumoniae 46
stressors 94–5
strongyloidosis 3
support groups
patients 96
staff 116
suramin 124

tears 34
tinea species 43
thromboccytopenia 41, 44, 49
thymus gland 28
toxoplasma gondii 32, 42, 46–7
toxoplasmosis 3, 46–7, 60
trimethoprim-sulfamethoxazole (co-
trimoxazole) 44–5, 77
triclosan 2% (Ster-Zac bath concentrate) 88

vaccine 126
varicella-zoster virus 16–17, 49
varicella (chickenpox) 17, 58
vinblastine 53
virion 13
virus
structure 12–14
progenitor agent of HIV 17
receptor sites 15
visitors 89, 92
visna virus 15

warts, genital 42
white blood cell count 24–5, 49

Zaire 17–18
zoster (shingles) 17, 42–3, 50, 59